WHAT THIS BOOK [   ] FOR YOU:

1. Help you understand why you awaken tired and stiff . . . why your back hurts when you sit, stand and walk . . . and what you must do to free yourself from pain.

2. Teach you to locate the root cause of back problems and how you must apply this knowledge to relieve your pain.

3. Wipe out your existing confusion about backache and replace it with the positive attitude leading to total, welcome relief.

4. Figuratively, hold-your-hand during an acute backache and sympathetically describe how to gain control over pain, anxiety and hopelessness.

5. Give you an appetizing list of solutions you must have to rid yourself of the habits and attitudes which create back pain.

6. Guide you to a brighter self-image through the magic of posture awareness and exercises which reward you with a balanced body and mind.

7. Demonstrate with 90 illustrations the methods proven by chiropractic physicans to solve backache without drugs or surgery.

8. Show how to benefit from taking responsibility for your own health . . . learn and apply action solutions. . . forego excuses and "over-the-backyard-fence" diagnosis and remedies.

9. Train you to live better, happier when you free yourself from back pain.

10. Make it possible to know what you must do for yourself — and with help from your doctor — to say Bye Bye Backache.

i

BYE BYE BACKACHE

David C. Lindsey, D.C.

d'Carlin Publishing
P.O. Box 534
Carlsbad, CA 92008

First Printing August, 1981
Second Printing April, 1983
Third Printing, June, 1986

Library of Congress Card Catalog No. 81-67080
ISBN: 0-939342-01-4

Printed in the United States of America

iv

Table of Contents

vi

ILLUSTRATIONS

FIGURE   **PAGE**

Preface

How do I know how you feel when you come to my office doubled over with cramps and pain? I've been there myself, down on the floor, hurting and helpless.

That is why I empathize with you—I know what you're thinking. I listen when you ask: "Doc, what's wrong with me? Will I ever be my old self again?"

"Why did this happen to me?" I hear you. Every patient wants the answer to his personal problem.

That's what this book is all about . . . how do backaches start? Why do they persist? How can they be eliminated? How can I help myself?

In my case, I was thirty-four before discovering my problem, a birth defect in my lower lumbar vertebra, a spondylolisthesis. By age fifty-four, I also discovered my low back and cervical area was loaded with arthritic deposits. One doctor pronounced judgment: I would have to stop practicing, it was too strenuous.

But, thanks to faith, exercise, nutrition and regular chiropractic adjustments, today, eleven years later, I'm in far better physical shape than the diagnostician, several years my junior.

Had someone told me I had a bad back before I entered high school, played football and entered into high springboard diving competition—working out five or more hours daily springing on the board and hitting the water, many times flat on my back—I could have been spared much pain and personal readjustment later in life. I wasn't told not to do certain things because my complaints were dismissed as "growing pains."

No one knew—or appeared to care—that I had a genuine and serious back problem . . . I looked pretty good and physical on the outside.

I later learned my father was discharged from the navy due to arthritis and that spondylolisthesis is frequently passed from father to son.

The lessons I've learned from academic training, trial-and-error and clinical experience that keep me going at a healthy clip . . . it's all in Bye Bye Backache . . . it can keep you going, too.

The basics are simple to master: 1) acknowledge that you have a problem 2) find competent help—from a professional source and from your new understanding of what's required of you and 3) believe with all your strength that *you can be helped.*

Bye Bye Backache directs you to the source of your problem. It offers specific exercises, nutritional advice and home-remedies that relieve back pain and joint stiffness.

This book honestly answers all your pertinent questions. It provides methods for correcting posture with simple exercises, which in thousands of cases, have strengthened supporting ligaments, muscle groups and tendons, eliminating backache. Countless documented cases found in the professional reference texts—Comroe's *Arthritis*, Goldthwait's *Essentials of Body Mechanics*, Jackson's *The Cervical Syndrome*, Calliet's *Soft Tissue Pain and Disability*, Kliner's *Human Biochemistry* and many others—are medical in their concepts. Therefore, it is gratifying to find abundant agreement with the drugless profession of chiropractic in the clinical application of posture correction—not medicine, not surgery—as a basic requirement for relief of backache and related musculo-skeletal conditions.

Today people seek an alternate method to drugs, and more personal attention to their problems for the relief of back pain and muscle tension, by-products of stress, modern lifestyles and cultural adaptations.

Is this the realization of Thomas Edison's turn-of-the-century prediction that "Doctors of the future will give no medicine but will interest his patient in the care of the human frame, in diet and the cause and prevention of disease?"

The fact that more people will receive this message—and find help for their personal ailments—through these printed words than is possible through person-to-person contact in the office makes this undertaking more worthwhile . . . it makes it indispensable in terms of improved over-all health at reduced cost.

There is an immense personal satisfaction knowing, at last, there is a complete source of reference for the desperate questions surrounding backache.

Thanks are deserved by the great number of chiropractic professionals who have enthusiastically supported this effort with their suggestions, advice, criticism and corrective exercises which they personally have proven in their offices.

Another group deserves thanks . . . the millions of chiropractic patients who have shared in telling others the benefits of chiropractic.

And my wife, Kathleen, who has freely given love and support.

David C. Lindsey, D.C.

CHAPTER 1
Balance: The Backache Stops Here

James is a retired Air Force Colonel and an usher at our church. For three years I watched with professional interest the strange way he walked up and down the aisle. He dragged his left foot. His back swayed from left to right. This Sunday he added a peculiar twist, a kind of Walter Brennan hitch. I couldn't stand it any longer. I cornered him during the coffee social hour following services.

"James," I said, "Come to my office this week...no excuses."

"Thanks, Doc, but I'm a helpless case. I walk funny because I've got a short leg."

James did visit me, twice. He left walking fairly normally for someone with one leg almost one inch shorter than the other. He didn't drag his foot. His back didn't sway. And, he had no pain in the sacro-iliac joint to compensate for.

He was fitted with pelvic stabilizers, a combination rubber and leather device which is worn inside each shoe. A cast was made of the feet and the inserts were designed and molded to shift the body weight back to a balanced foundation. They also were shaped to move the center of gravity back to the proper level of the spine. James became balanced.

Surprised? That equalizing James' leg lengths and restoring balance eased his backache? Can this same solution — rebalancing — also free you from back pain?

Yes. Practically all structural backache will improve in relation to the return of balance.

Our Universe — and everything in it — is subject to balance. It's not the exclusive property of mankind. Environmental coexistence with the forces of gravity demands it. We must have balance to function at maximum efficiency.

It's established that imbalance on a major scale, resulting in death and destruction to millions of people, can occur from a slight shift in the rotational axis of the earth. This deviation from normal balance can set off a series of violent volcanic eruptions along the entire volcanic chain.

Will thinking in terms of "cosmic togetherness" or "environmental harmony" make it easier to accept an overall concept of how important balance is to life? However viewed, the reality is this: Becoming balanced means losing your backache. And, that's what this book is all about.

Glancing briefly at history may present a clearer picture of why backache seems to accompany our cultural progression.

Long ago, before the luxury of THE MACHINE, Man accomplished physical tasks with the handiest tool available, his own body. He stooped, squatted, bent, tugged, pulled, hauled, scooped, split trees and quarried rocks — all the hard way. We can believe this activity created a body of awesome physical proportions. And, it's reasonable to believe, it also produced some awful backaches, too.

Would this be Man's first medical problem? Back strain?

We learn that he sought relief in a variety of ways. One crudely effective remedy was having a bear walk on his "sore back."

As culture flowered so did the medical sophistication in dealing with spinal stress. Practitioners, each in their own fashion, ran the gamut of ready cures. They explained to Man the nature of his problem to suit the context of the current cultural mode: "It's due to the air, vapors, thick and thin blood, the curse-of-the-year, guts, food, miasma, flux, elimination, "something that needs cutting out of your body", demons or crazy notions in the head, or the result of your own evil doing.

Presumably, over the years all the attending witches, gods and medicine men did some good because man persists in consulting the "experts" for relief of back pain. However, history records that with the appearance of science, as we recognize it today, and the advent of moon-walking technology, Man still suffers an old-fashioned garden variety of backache.

We no longer attach familiar names to it, like lumbago or rheumatism. Backache comes to you today with the communicative jelly of Madison Avenue; tenosinovitis, sciatica, facet syndrome, degenerative disc disease, fibrositis, and psychosomatic illness. Nevertheless, to the person who has — or gets — pain in the back, there's not a better expression to describe this complaint than BACKACHE.

It's not a solitary malady. Backache is shared non-exclusively by millions the world over without regard for sex, age or money-in-the-bank. It strikes anytime, any place. Its effects are universally torturous.

Well, now you are aware that your specific disorder occupies a significant role in medical history and literature, what, you want to know, can be done for it?

You can help yourself by taking two giant steps forward:

3

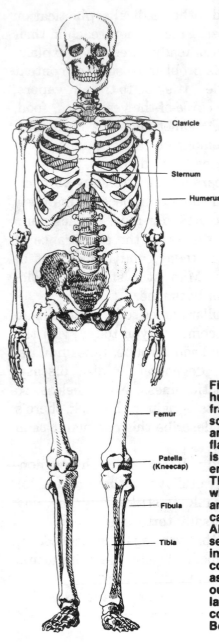

Clavicle

Sternum

Humerus

Femur

Patella
(Kneecap)

Fibula

Tibia

Fig. 1—The 206 bones of the human skeleton provide the framework for attachment of the soft tissues of the body. There are various types of bone: long, flat, oval, etc. The most common is the long bone, with the knobby ends and tapering middle shaft. The ends of bone (the epiphyses) which forms a movable joint with another bone, is covered with cartilage to prevent friction. Also, bones in a joint may be separated by a cartilage disc, as in the vertebra of the spinal column, or a miniscus cartilage as in the knee. Inside the hard outer layer of bone is a nutritive lattice-work of canals which contain bone marrow and blood. Bones harden with aging. Sur-

4

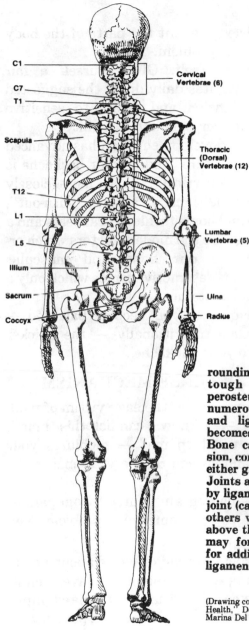

C1

Cervical
Vertebrae (6)

C7

T1

Scapula

Thoracic
(Dorsal)
Vertebrae (12)

T12

L1

L5

Lumbar
Vertebrae (5)

Illium

Sacrum

Ulna

Coccyx

Radius

rounding the exterior of bone is a tough fibrous coating, the perosteum, to which are attached numerous blood vessels, tendons and ligaments. This covering becomes less vascular with aging. Bone can withstand more tension, compression and shear than either granite or white oak.

Joints are maintained in position by ligaments which surround the joint (capsular ligaments) and by others which attach to the bone above the bone below. They also may form a criss-cross pattern for additional strength (cruciate ligaments).

(Drawing courtesy of John Thie, D.C., "Touch for Health," De Vorss & Co., 1046 Princeton Dr., Marina Del Rey, CA 90291)

5

1. Gain more knowledge about the parts of the body involved in your specific problem.
2. Cooperate with yourself. Give yourself a fair chance. Spend a few minutes daily doing the suggested exercises to relieve tension and stress to sensitive tissues, the sources of your pain and disability.

Over the years of our development Man has advanced physically to Modern Culture. Today your backache is seldom the cause of "overwork". It is more closely associated with the conditions of stress, "burn-out", coping, wicked office and home furniture, car seats and a terrible mattress. These are the modern factors which orchestrate imbalance to our bony and muscular framework. These are the destructive forces which only a return to balance can counteract.

Consequently, the quicker you become balanced — physically, mentally and nutritionally — the quicker you'll say Bye Bye to your backache.

MOBILIZE YOUR DEFENSE MECHANISM

Negative thinking makes you the easy victim of pain.

Thinking positively — "I know I can lick this thing", "I know the doctor will help me" — mobilizes your defense mechanism and speeds recovery. It makes the juices flow.

You can unlearn — deprogram yourself from pain — with a strong desire to overcome your problem. You have the power.

How many times have you read or heard about a frail woman actually lifting an automobile to save a child trapped beneath the wheels? This is an extreme example of the power of concentration. It's an act of a person who

6

takes a positive action rather than be a party to a tragedy because the outcome is not predetermined. You can't judge the outcome of your actions unless you take them. And, when you do, play the game to win.

Accomplish your game plan by believing you can be helped.

Know you can conquer your symptoms. Lead yourself, don't allow pain to control your thinking. Take command! This action by itself will mobilize every defense mechanism in your body.

The millions of cells circulating in your bloodstream behave like tiny slaves; they obey your every command. So, command them. Make them heal you, not hurt you. You, and you alone, must make them know what you expect of them.

It may be easier if you challenge yourself. Make a game of your own invention.

You learn to subdue your annoying mechanical defect by unlearning the improper habits of body mechanics. This book can teach you how. Isn't that the reason you bought it? To get rid of your backache?

COMMON ORIGINS OF BACK PAIN

Most frequently, pain in the back originates, or is associated with, a combination of factors which result in structural/mechanical/postural imbalance.

One side of the body is on the receiving end of symptoms related to imbalance, decrease in normal nerve energy to local tissues, poor circulation/nutrition, build-up of toxic waste products (catabolites), irritation,

7

inflammation, swelling, shorter range-of-motion, unusual shearing pressure and joint friction, plus non-reversible, abnormal wear on the cartilage and bony surface of the joint.

Weakness in an individual or group of muscles on one side of the body causes the spine to curve toward the side of weakness. This stretches the muscle attachments of the opposite side, causing them to become tight, knotty and irritable. Also the supporting ligaments are overly stretched, making it difficult to hold the skeletal structure in erect alignment. This is demonstrated in the illustrations shown in Figs. 2, 3, 4, and 5.

You can recognize these conditions in others quite easily. One hip is higher than the other, the head tilts to one side, one shoulder-blade protrudes or one shoulder is higher than the opposite side.

An imbalanced condition also affects joints other than the back. The identical set of circumstances may account for joint pain in the knee, shoulder, arm or leg. All healing professions agree in this basic concept.

Correcting the majority of spinal ailments begins with an analysis of the posture (Fig. 6).

The examiner looks for the area of imbalance. Following this appraisal, the program for correction is aimed directly at the pain-producing tissues located at the sites of imbalance. The original cause of your symptoms may be the result of an accident (Fig. 7), occupational stress or habitual bad posture leading to overuse, disuse or premature wearing-out of bone structure or a change in the normal composition of tissue fibers.

Regardless of cause, relief comes by removing irritation from the offending tissues surrounding the

8

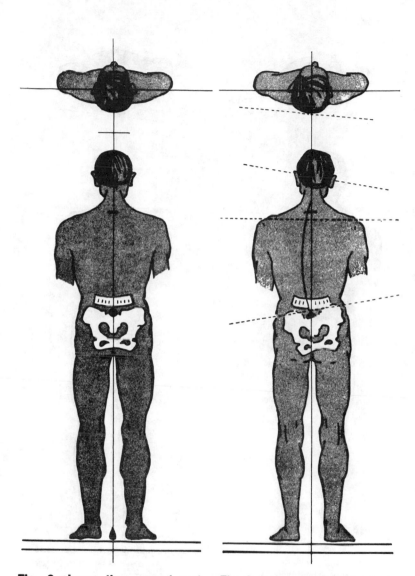

Fig. 2 shows the normal and balanced posture, back view. The skeletal muscles are in balance on both sides of the body.

Fig. 3 demonstrates a weakness of the left muscles in the lower and middle back.

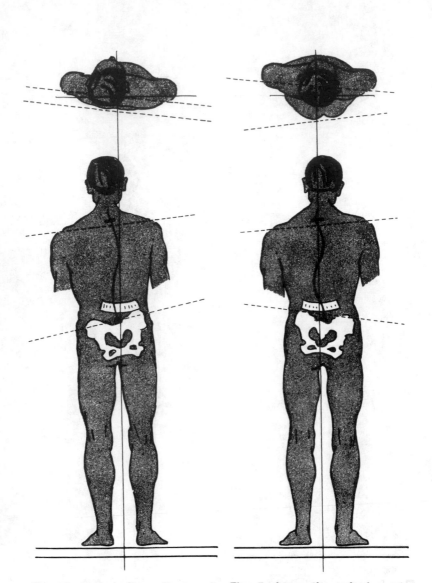

Fig. 4 shows the effects of weakness in muscles in the left low back and right middle areas of the spine.
(Drawings courtesy of Fred Stoner D.C., author of "The Eclectic Approach to Chiropractic," F.L.S. Publishing Co., Las Vegas, Nevada.)

Fig. 5 shows the spinal curves associated with muscle weakness in the right lower back and right middle back. Note how the entire body tends to turn toward the side of weakness.

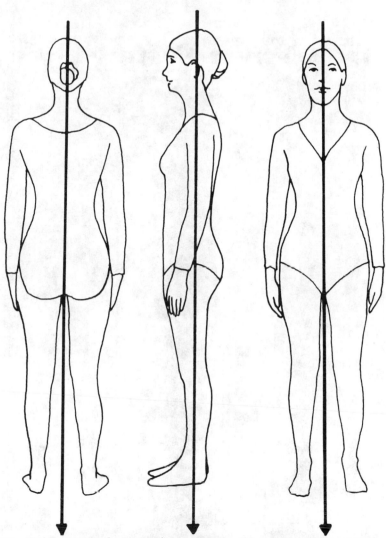

Fig. 6A An example of perfect posture. To analyze your posture,
visualize a vertical line that runs through the ear . . . through the
shoulder . . . midway through the chest . . . through the hip . . . through
the knee . . . and through the ankle. This is the role-model children
should adopt to develop their posture. When begun early in life, good
posture becomes a fixed habit. Every home and classroom should
display a Perfect Posture Chart to train children in this important
aspect of body and health development. Every adult should use the
Perfect Posture Chart daily to gain awareness of healthful benefits of
improved posture.

11

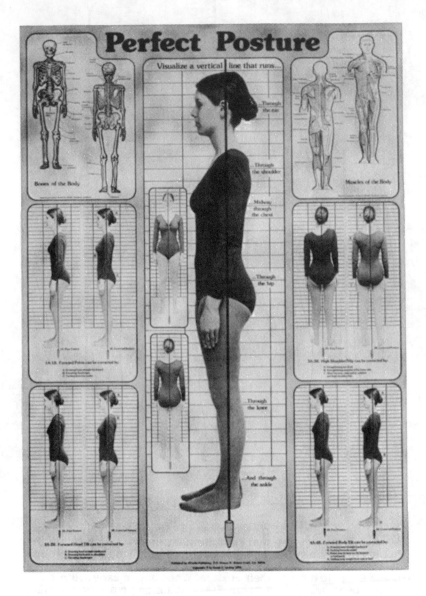

Fig. 6B—The perfect posture chart.

12

Fig. 7 shows the effects of a muscle spasm on the lower (lumbar) spine. The contraction of heavy muscles in this area pulls the lumbar spine backward, "flattening" the customary curve (lordosis) in this area. This is a defensive mechanism of the body, to "splint" the area to protect against further damage. This alteration in normal spinal alignment may also produce some pressure at the bottom verterbra (Fifth Lumbar) where it sits atop the sacrum, the tail-bone.

imbalanced areas, whether occurring in the spine, shoulders or extremities.

Posture is our upright position in standing, sitting or moving. Imbalance may occur in four directions: front, back, left or right. Or at a downward slant, as with the pregnant female, who adopts a waddling, duck-like gait.

A sideward (lateral) spinal curve may result from continual contraction and/or development of muscle groups on one side of the body, or from repeated one-sided actions required in sports or certain occupations. Spinal tilting may also result from weak muscles.

Golf, tennis and racquetball tend to overdevelop one side of the body, as do occupations like operating a punch press. Both conditions lead to an overall condition of imbalance.

Another cause for imbalance is loss of the normal elasticity in ligaments and in the spinal discs through aging, injury or constant misuse.

The ends of bone are shaped to allow for a specific pattern of motion, such as the full movement of a finger joint or the very slight gliding motion of the collarbone. When body weight and unusual pressure on a joint causes uneven wear, the bone will change its shape and conform to the direction of the pressure. A usually wedge-shaped vertebra may even become pie-shaped, resulting from poor standing or sitting posture.

Uneven bone wear at the joint surface may cause the the shock-absorbing disc to carry too much pressure on the side of exceptional contact. This results in wearing out or degeneration of the disc and a condition called osteo-arthritis.

The muscle fibers which attach to the bone surface now may be altered in their ordinary tension, causing irritation and spasm.

The ligaments also may be affected at their normal points of attachment, and disturbing their customary function may cause them to lose their fluid content, consequently, lose their normal elasticity, making it easier to strain the back at this specific level of limited joint movement.

EMOTIONS AFFECT YOUR
CHEMICAL BALANCE

The above factors, which influence normal skeletal balance, are subject indirectly, to your emotional behavior.

Fear, anger, anxiety and depression cause reactions which adversely affect the naturally harmonious relationships within the "total" body.

Fear constricts the blood vessels, dilates the pupils, moves blood from the organs to the external muscles, increases blood pressure and breathing, releases adrenalin into the bloodstream and, in general, produces an over-all attitude of Fight or Flight. This is known as Sympathetic Dominance and will be discussed in more detail in Chapters 2 and 4.

These stress-producing and tension-related ingredients, which are chemical in nature as well as physical, can overwhelm you with a powerful, negative effect upon the tissues which trigger the irritation recognized as backache.

No matter which occurs first, the physical or emotional stimulus...both initiating sources of pain mean trouble.

Either emotional or musculoskeletal irritants—both may start imbalance to the sensitive cycle of secretion within the internal glandular system. An upsetting influence excites the adrenal glands which sit atop the kidneys and produce adrenalin.

This powerful chemical is antagonistic to insulin, a chemical substance produced by the pancreas gland which functions to maintain a normal level of sugar in the blood.

Adrenalin causes a rise in blood sugar. However, when an unusually high blood sugar level is quickly decreased, muscles may cramp and gastric and elimination systems are disturbed. Over-stimulation of the adrenal glands result in fatigue and chronic imbalance in the circulating blood sugar levels.

A low level of sugar in the bloodstream (hypoglycemia) affects the mental processes and disrupts rhythmic muscular movements, replacing smoothness with jerky, erratic behavior.

The by-products of glandular imbalance may be hyperkinetic behavior (spastic, uneven muscle contractions, excessive fatigue, emotional irritability and finally, coma).

The brain itself is divided and subject to imbalance between its right and left portions. Presently, investigations are being made into functions of each separate area of the brain. Much of this revealing research concerns matching specific behavior to either right or left cranial locations. This will be discussed in more detail in Chapter 4.

BALANCE RELATES TO FUNCTION

One word sums up the basic requirement for a full, active life: Balance.

My great-grandfather used to talk about one aspect of

balance like this: "Eat when you're hungry; drink when you're dry." His point was to avoid excess and to live life in moderation.

Good health is actually good balance, essentially between extremes. Technically, balance is a condition called "homeostasis," equilibrium between different but interdependent elements of a group.

Loss of balance results in loss of function.

You can measure your loss of function by recognizing the absence, rather than the presence, of certain physical activities.

The greater the loss, the more severe the illness.

A backache, as nobody need tell you, lowers your ability to function at 100% efficiency. You may be conditioned to believe being half-alive is all you can expect of yourself, but this is absolutely untrue.

Withdrawal is the usual pattern.

You've stopped playing; you won't compete. You walk rather than run. You avoid the simple pleasurable activities—gardening, building or taking long drives during vacation. Perhaps you're fearful of playing with small children, lifting furniture or making the necessary body movements in your favorite sport or recreational activity.

When you can bend, stoop or squat only so far because pain puts on the brakes, you can be sure that a return to balance can correct this condition and restore your health.

You should be able to stand, sit, walk and sleep in any position you wish without pain or restriction.

There's a solution for every problem.

Some individuals understand the working of an auto better than they do their own body. They are capable of making simple adjustments to solve difficulties. When a wheel of their car is out of balance (alignment) they immediately place a 50¢ lead weight to it and correct this problem, which, uncorrected, may cause premature wearing out of the tire.

A different person, one who understands the body, may recognize that his back pain is due to one leg being shorter than the other. This condition tilts the pelvis and causes pain in the back, possibly in the sacro-iliac joint. A 75¢ heel lift placed in the shoe of the short leg can correct this imbalance. With both legs even, pain leaves the back, endurance is increased and reluctance to join the fun with the sports gang is gone forever.

SHOES PROVIDE CLUES OF IMBALANCE

How do you recognize spinal imbalance?

Look at your feet. Body imbalance begins there.

A quick examination of your shoes might reveal uneven wear, a certain indication of body imbalance. One heel may wear down faster than the other, either on the inside or outside (Fig. 8). Uneven sole wear on either side or at the toe shows unevenness and erratic foot or leg movement. If your shoes show uneven wear, repair or replace them before starting the exercises and programs suggested in this book.

Your shoes now become an instrument to measure your progress, a witness to your return to a balanced state.

Other signs of imbalance deliver a more painful message. Muscle cramping, shooting pain associated

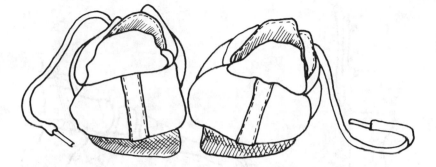

Fig. 8—An example of shoes run-down on the outside. If one side of your shoe is worn more than the opposite, you have the evidence of your body imbalance.

with certain body movement, nausea, headache, fatigue and pelvic dysfunction are signals which disappear when muscles are no longer required to do the work designed for ligaments and when the muscle strength is evenly divided between the right and left sides of your body.

THE ROLE OF FEET IN POSTURE

Postural imbalance tends to move upward from the foot, through the ankle and knee, to the hip and spine and ends at the head. Knowing this, you may not be surprised to learn a headache can be triggered from a remote source, such as the feet (Fig. 9).

Abnormal tissue growth on the feet—callouses, corns and bunions—contribute to malalignment in your architectural structure. Birth defects, such as irregular toe formation and weak arch development also cause the

19

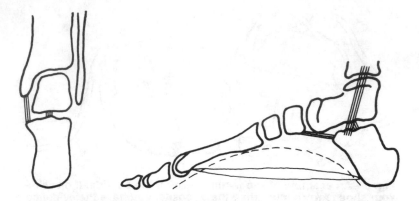

Fig. 9—Shows the normal foot alignment from the rear view. B) The well-formed longitudinal arch. Deviation in this arch can cause a shift in body weight which results in faulty posture.

erect body posture to shift into an imbalanced attitude.

Certainly, if your foundation is off-level, your roof will be, too. A house wouldn't stand long with this engineering imperfection and, while you might not be blown down by a strong wind, you'll most certainly suffer the consequences of poor structural design...and suffer some degree of pain along the way (Fig. 10).

Ankle, knee and hip pain may be directly related to mechanical defects in the postural foundation, the feet (Fig. 11).

Biochemical imbalance causes an inventory of unwanted physical symptoms, from loss of normal range-of-motion and irregular muscle movement and rhythm to deviation from normal physiological and psychological responses. Your health quotient is below the level expected of your age and physical development. And, chances are, your overall thinking patterns, social behavior and work performances are beneath your potential.

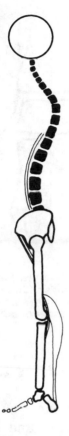

Fig. 10—Correct erect stance is maintained primarily by the ligaments. Very little muscle support is needed with good posture. Only with imbalance are the muscles called upon to take over the normal function of ligaments. When this occurs, the body becomes fatigued from excessive muscle exertion.

You have the power and ability to change this inventory of spinal imbalance. The solution seems too simple to accept easily. All that's required is for you to broaden your perspective to accept the clear fact that your problem is related to physical, emotional and/or chemical distortion.

Sure, a pill may deaden your sensibilities temporarily, but it won't correct your imbalance or remove forever the cause of your discomfort. The final solution rests with you.

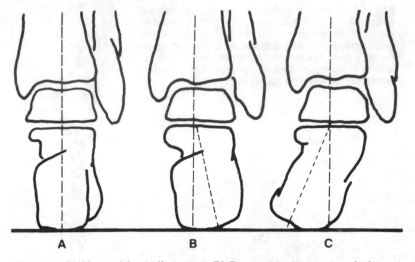

Fig. 11—A) Normal foot alignment. B) Demonstrates uneven balance causing shifting of weight to the mid-line. This is known as pronation. C) A weight shift to the outside is known as supination. Both of these abnormal conditions can painfully affect the entire spinal structure.

GRAVITY INDUCED SPINAL ADJUSTMENTS

Physical balance requires good posture in standing, walking and sitting. It must be practiced every day, every hour of the day, not just when fatigue or a stab of pain reminds us to change positions. An erect stance must be maintained continually to overcome the force of gravity, which exerts a constant downward pull on our body.

Balance requires adequate muscle tone throughout the body—the front as well as the back—and sufficient bilateral strength to prevent tilting of the head, shoulder or hip to the side of weakness. As you progress through the chapters of this book, you'll better understand how a little bit of poor posture becomes exaggerated more each day at the expense of supporting tissues which must bear the burden of your imbalance.

Over eons changes have occurred in the human spine, due partly to the decline in heavy, stoop labor and food gathering customs.

At birth the spine is without curves. As the infant gains strength in the neck from attempting to hold up its head, the *cervical* curve is formed. Low back muscles develop from standing erect and form the lowest *(lumbar)* curve. The mid-back curve forms as a balance between these two curves.

Spinal curves allow the upright body to absorb the shock of compression and achieve upright balance against gravity.

Obviously, increasing or decreasing the depth of any of these three curves shifts the ideal center of gravity forward or backward, causing an unwanted and

Fig. 12—The progress of the human spine, from infancy (A) through adulthood (B). The three curves of the spine occur as the infant develops strength to hold up the head (cervical lordosis), then the second curve (lumbar lordosis) appears as we overcome additional gravitational force. The curve in the mid-spine, the dorsal kyphosis, gives overall balance between the upper and lower portions of the spine.

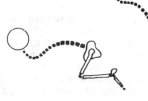

A   B

subconscious bending of the trunk to maintain balance (Fig. 13).

If you are causing a sway-back by bending backward to overcome extra weight in the abdominal area, you are moving your center of gravity away from its proper axis. You're creating an imbalanced structure, which is like writing the first painful chapter in your own book of backache.

Pain results from irritation to certain tissues in the

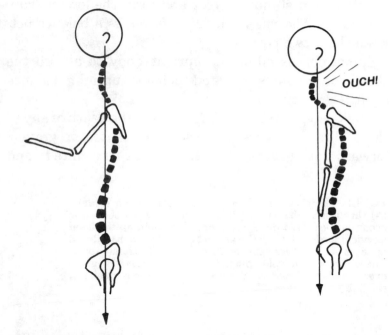

Fig. 13—How faulty posture causes pain in the neck. Carrying the head downward of the proper center of gravity causes the shoulders to fall forward and downward and the mid-back to bend backward into a kyphosis. This attitude is the typical slouched position. It causes downward pressure on the diaphragm and reduced capacity in the lungs. This common postural fault can be responsible for shoulder and neck pain. Continual forward head carrage can result in degeneration of the cervical disc and low back pain due to forward dropping of the pelvis.

specific area of imbalance. In addition, nerve impulses may transmit these undesirable sensations to other sectors of the body. You may trigger pain to reflex areas of pain in other parts of the body. This is motivation enough for practicing correct posture.

It's the price you must pay to stop your backache.

THE PRICE OF PAIN

Can one put a price on a backache?

To become accomplished at anything requires practice. Actors must act. Musicians must play. Athletes must work out.

To expect relief from pain, you must practice better posture all day long, not just when you hurt. Doing this will reduce strain, friction, stress, tension and irritation to helpless tissues.

Try measuring your cost for relief in terms of the amount of time spent to accomplish good balance. This has to be the best health bargain you'll ever find.

One of my most outstanding accomplishments in many years of treating backache was with Mary, who made the swiftest recovery of any patient within my memory.

"There's only one way to get rid of your pelvic pain, Mary ..." I was very firm. "Stop wearing those super-high-heeled pumps."

Of course she didn't want to forsake fashion for comfort. What young, attractive lady does? But, losing days every month from work, plus the necessity of frequently making excuses to "favor" her back pain, gave Mary the motivation she needed to change to more practical footwear.

I saw her recently at a football game. She was wearing tight jeans and the most outrageously high pair of heels I'd ever seen.

"Oh, Doctor, I haven't had a symptom in months. Don't scold me about my shoes. I only wear them now on special occasions." Well, I guess half a loaf is better than no bread at all.

Mary's cost to cure backache wasn't very expensive. But, whether you find relief as fast as Mary or much more slowly, the price is the same for everyone... adjusting the offending cause and returning to a state of balance. Put what you learn into action, this will keep the price you must pay at a minimum.

GAIN AWARENESS FROM THE PERFECT POSTURE MODEL

The Perfect Posture Chart (Fig. 6) shows how easy it is to follow a visual model. Have someone check your posture from the front, side and back. Will a plumb line dissect you through the ear, shoulder, midway through the chest, the hip and ankle?

Does it require tension to duplicate the Posture model? Good posture makes you look good, relaxed and it transmits a strong, robust feeling.

If your first glance at the model reveals errors in your posture and it prompts you to "straighten up" as best you presently know how, that's great! But, imagine how much more productive a large wall chart, 24" x 36", can be. We urge you to have this Perfect Posture Chart on your wall at home so you can see it every day. (Available from D'Carlin Publishing, P.O. Box 534, Carlsbad, CA, 92008 at $9.95 plus $1.00 postage).

One wall in every home, classroom, office and factory should display the message expressed in the Perfect Posture Chart for one compelling reason: it promotes AWARENESS. This is the ingredient lacking where it is needed the most, where we work or play and where we learn (mainly by repetition). We benefit from the forces of gravity to remain erect and balanced.

There's no free lunch.

Good health carries a price tag. The price you pay to conquer backache is directly proportionate to your desire to be free of pain. The more frequently you practice good posture, the faster you'll experience relief. The more positive you think the less pain you are bound to encounter. All in all, a pretty fair return, wouldn't you agree, for this investment in yourself?

LOVE YOURSELF—YOU'RE ALL YOU'VE GOT

Not everyone is alike, either in physical or emotional constitution or in their response to pain and other stimuli.

Briefly, there are three different recognizable body types: slender, stocky and medium, midway between slender and stocky. Each of these distinct body builds (Fig. 14) is as different as fingerprints on your thumb. Since you're genetically bound to follow the disposition

27

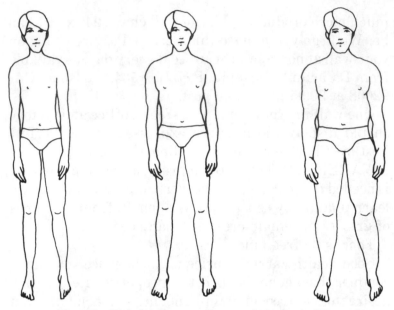

Fig. 14—The slender, medium and stocky builds.

of your particular body construction, it makes good sense to love yourself—as your are—and correct whatever weakness exists. You're all you've got, there's no starting over from scratch.

THE SLENDER TYPE

The slender type with a relatively small and short intestine, can handle a concentrated diet. The muscles are small in bulk and the extremities are tapering and long. The feet are narrow with a high arch. The joints have a loose ligamentous attachment and the range of motion may be 15-30% greater than that of a stocky type. The torso is longer and narrower with a greater tendency for the abdominal organs to sag (Fig. 15). The

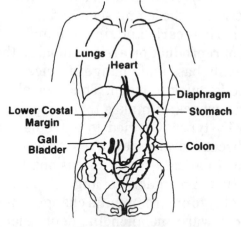

The Slender Type

Fig. 15—The slender type, 35% of the community, has a greater tendency of abdominal sag. This can be responsible for constipation and other digestive disturbances.

spine is lighter and more slender, and there is a predisposition to having an extra vertebra, a sixth lumbar, for example. The lungs are smaller in area and the heart is positioned more in the mid-portion of the chest. The stomach is long and tubular with longer attachments. The large intestine is from three to five feet shorter in the slender type.

The slender type usually has low blood pressure and is prone to acute type of illness rather than chronic disease. The body inclines backward from the low lumbar region increasing the lumbar *lordosis* and forward inclination of the pelvis, tending to cause increased roundness of the mid and upper dorsal region. This also encourages a forward projection of the head and neck. The chest is flattened, decreasing the vital capacity of the lungs. The knees may be *hyperextended* causing a pronation of the feet with strain on the leg muscles and arches of the foot.

Puberty arrives early and, in the female, problems in the organs of reproduction are common. In the male, the voice is usually bass and change of voice comes early.

This type is quick to learn. This special quality may have one drawback: it makes them impatient with the slower stocky types. Carried to extremes, the slender type may become overly devoted to "causes," tending to become dogmatical, and, occasionally, fanatical. Although they are quick to anger, the slender type adjusts quickly to environmental changes. He or she may be inclined toward melancholia, depression and acute nervous and mental disorders. Slender persons generally are introverted and self-conscious.

THE STOCKY TYPE

The stocky type has a long intestine, perhaps twenty feet more than the slender type. The limbs are large and heavy and the muscle fibers are coarser and less elastic. Range of motion is usually 10-20 degrees less than normal. The foot arch is low and the legs are shorter. There is an excess of fat throughout the body which may be associated with connective tissue, making the flesh firm and hard. The ribs are broad and heavy, more horizontal than those of the slender person, whose ribs slant downward. The lumbar spine is short and deep set between the *ilia*. The body cavities are larger and deeper. The intestinal organs are bigger and have shorter attachments, making sag a less common complaint

(Fig. 16). Backache develops much later in life since the general structure of the body withstands strain much better. However, as body weight increases in both the child and the adult, there occurs a backward inclination of the spine and *thorax* (chest) on the pelvis. Deformities are not common and develop later in life.

Passage of food through the alimentary system is slower in the stocky type, therefore the diet should be less concentrated as a longer time is permitted for digestion absorption and assimilation. The stocky type is more adapted to sustained action periods.

The even-tempered and easy-going stocky type get along well socially. They have a good sense of humor and are tolerant. They work more slowly, but have greater endurance and recover more slowly from fatigue than the slender type. They are not self-conscious and tend to

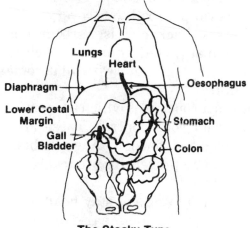

The Stocky Type

Fig. 16—The stocky type has less tendency to sag internal organs and diameter of colon is larger than the slender type.

be extroverts, however, they do not adjust easily to changes in their environment. They are not susceptible to acute disease, but suffer more from chronic ailments.

RECOGNIZE THE LIMITATIONS OF SELF-TREATMENT

No book on self-help is, or should be, taken as a substitute for qualified professional care. The fact is, you can gain much by receiving a thorough checkup from a chiropractor who will see that you're started on the right track with your personal rebuilding program.

You must learn to position your body precisely to reap the greatest benefit from the application of correct body mechanics. Once you've gained the knack and you can imitate the Perfect Posture model without outside help, you'll be far down the road to recovery.

In some cases, backache is a recurring condition caused by spinal malalignment which requires a chiropractic adjustment before it will become stabilized and symptom-free.

There are other conditions which become irritated due to factors beyond your control. These are commonly related to stress and tension. A workable solution in these cases may be a preventive program of chiropractic adjustments.

It makes excellent sense to stay healthy.

Achieving a state of near-perfect balance—homeostasis—has a price tag, as you've discovered. Only *you* can reestablish your body balance sufficiently to get rid of backache. Consequently, *you* have to make the decision to change *your* body—and pay the price by learning and maintaining good posture—by practicing specific exercises which restore balance to the entire muscle system.

Figs. 17 and 18 show several common bad postural habits, any of which can lead to painful spinal disability. Make every effort to find new ways to position your body to avoid tissue strain and tension.

In the next chapter you'll learn which of the body tissues are the cause of your back pain.

This recognition will be another positive step leading to a final elimination of backache.

While your new-found emphasis on balance will protect you and reduce your frequency of back and joint pain, it is important to recognize the specific behavior of the tissues affected by the problem which provokes your backache.

The following chapter reveals how to accurately locate the source of your pain and how to recognize which tissue—bone, muscles, ligament, nerve or blood vessel— is involved in the pain producing process.

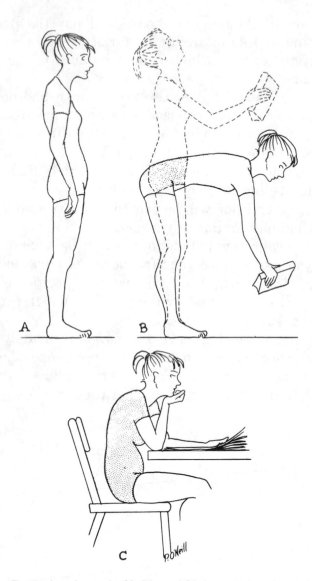

Fig. 17—Examples shown in A), B), and C) demonstrate how postural habits acquired at home or at work can cause repeated minor injury to the joints of the neck. Repeated irritation can inflame the nerve root, causing pain in the neck, shoulders and arms.

34

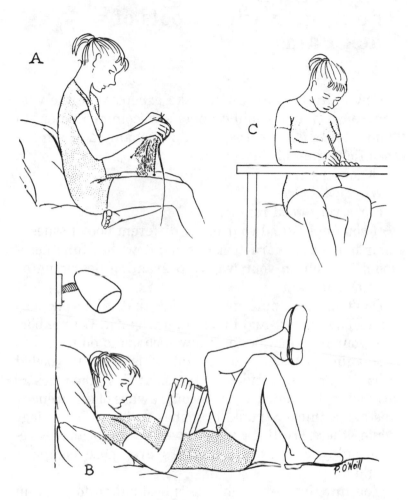

Fig. 18—While Fig. 17 shows a habitual backward bending of the neck, this shows the opposite, a constant habit of forward neckbending. While it seems harmless, constant irritation on the neck vertebra can result in permanent damage to the nerves and spinal discs, contributing to discomfort of headache, numbness and tingling in the arms and shoulder weakness.

(Figs. 17 and 18 courtesy of The Cervical Syndrome, Ruth Jackson, M.D., Published by Charles C Thomas, Springfield, Ill.

35

CHAPTER 2
The Aggravating Roots of Back Pain

Few chiropractors would take exception to the wisdom of a famous philosopher's recommendation to "know thyself!". Yet they would probably add a more specific urging of their own:

"Know thy tissues!"

Why?

For a very good reason.

If you understand your many different body tissues—their make-up, characteristics and how they function—you'll be well on your way to preventing, lessening or eliminating pain.

Don't for a minute get the idea that all tissues are alike. They're not, and I'll explain why not. Let me borrow your imagination for a few seconds to do it.

Imagine yourself walking into this heavily wooded area. You're surrounded by trees. At first, the trees all look alike, but quickly you become aware of differences: one has a thicker trunk, branches sprout spiny foliage while others are thick with leaves, fallen branches reveal pulpy centers while others are more compact, tougher.

You imagine how each tree is best suited for certain purposes if you were to cut them and build a house. The soft redwood with its colorful patterns would be perfect for the exterior. The tall pines would be more accessible and suitable for the framework, the studs.

Like trees in the forest, which seem alike, each of your body tissues is distinct. Each tissue reflects its indi-

36

vidual properties, fitting into the grand scheme of man's composition.

To pinpoint the root cause of your backache means putting the anatomical blame on the exact tissue or structure responsible for your particular problem.

Back pain can be traced to any one of the several tissues on the skeletal framework of the spinal column. It can be a muscle, ligament, tendon, blood vessel, nerve, bone, or a cartilagenous disc. Or, a combination of several tissues.

The following example makes this basic concept easy to understand.

Bone is hard and unyielding while the spinal disc is elastic with a movable pulpy interior; yet both can be responsible for the broad symptom of backache.

The blame must be put on the offending tissue before treatment will be meaningful in terms of saying "Bye Bye Backache." The chart shown in Fig. 19 presents a schematic cycle of the body and its progression to a final stage of backache.

To overcome your backache, treatment must be designed to reach and counteract the ill effects of the *actual* tissue producing your difficulty ... there's no panacea, no shotgun method which scatters soothing benefits to all tissues with equal effectiveness.

Gaining the skill to recognize your distress is the purpose of this book; however, a mistaken diagnosis can be unrewarding, as the following case demonstrates.

Peggy, bitterly disappointed when she first consulted me, was convinced nothing could be done to quiet the burning pain between her shoulder blades.

"I've just had three months of regular massage treatments," she said. "Today I don't feel any differently than

37

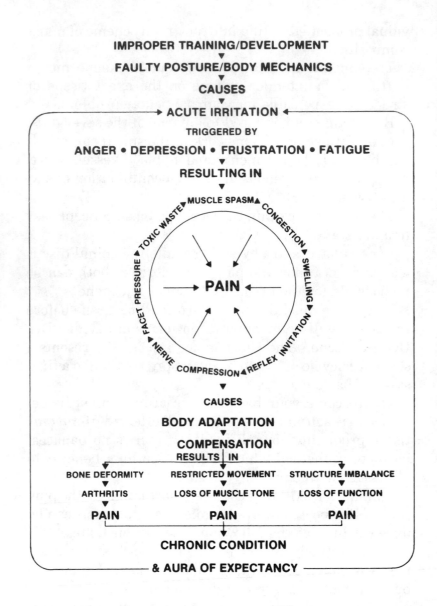

IMPROPER TRAINING/DEVELOPMENT
▼
FAULTY POSTURE/BODY MECHANICS
▼
CAUSES
▼
ACUTE IRRITATION

TRIGGERED BY

ANGER • DEPRESSION • FRUSTRATION • FATIGUE
▼
RESULTING IN
▼

MUSCLE SPASM
TOXIC WASTE
CONGESTION
FACET PRESSURE
SWELLING
PAIN
NERVE COMPRESSION
REFLEX INVITATION

▼
CAUSES
▼
BODY ADAPTATION
▼
COMPENSATION
RESULTS IN

BONE DEFORMITY	RESTRICTED MOVEMENT	STRUCTURE IMBALANCE
▼	▼	▼
ARTHRITIS	LOSS OF MUSCLE TONE	LOSS OF FUNCTION
▼	▼	▼
PAIN	**PAIN**	**PAIN**

CHRONIC CONDITION

& AURA OF EXPECTANCY

Fig. 19

before taking these treatments."

It was the truth. Her treatments accomplished no lasting relief because they were applied to the wrong tissues. Massage is helpful for muscle conditions; they do not affect the positioning of bones in the spine.

Peggy's case had been misdiagnosed.

Her difficulty was a malalignment—a *subluxation*— of a vertebra in the mid-spine area. The x-ray showed the problem. No wonder massage had no lasting value in overcoming her backache while a chiropractic adjustment did.

The proper treatment—and correct diagnosis—for Peggy was directed at the bone, the root cause of her distress.

Becoming familiar with the substance, workings and habits of various body tissues will help you discover the clues leading to the roots of your aggravation.

THE BONES

There are 206 bones in your body. Twenty-six, roughly are located in the spinal column: 7 in the neck (*cervical*); 12 in the mid-spine (*thoracic*); 6 in the lower back (*lumbar*). The *sacrum* and at its tip, the *coccyx*, form the "tailbone," the lowest segments of the spine.

You have 12 ribs, 6 on each side, which connect to the vertebra in the back and the breastbone, the sternum, in the front.

See the illustration of the skeleton in Chapter 1 (Fig.1).

Bone receives its nourishment from its outer-most coating, the *periosteum*. If this is damaged by injury,

39

the bone suffers, even dies, from lack of adequate nutrition. Extreme vascular congestion near bone can shut off the normal flow of life-sustaining nutrients to the bone. Bone marrow fills the cavities of bone, the site of red blood cell production. The body's defensive army of white cells also are manufactured and housed within the inner canals of bone.

JOINTS OF THE BODY

A joint is the location where bones join together. With movable joints, the bony surfaces are covered with tough padding, called *elastic fibrocartilages*, such as a spinal disc separating individual vertebra of the spine. There may be a thin sac of lubricating fluid between joints called *synovial fluid*. A joint may be further strengthened by strong fibrous bands of ligaments between bones forming a joint.

A joint functions much like a hinge to allow movement in the bony framework, and, like a hinge, restricts movements to a given distance, called *range-of-motion* (ROM). When a joint bends beyond its capacity (ROM) immediate damage results. As an example, a strain/sprain injury can result in torn ligaments and muscle attachments, ruptured *synovial sacs* with dischage of fluid, leaving the joint dry, and damage to the *periosteal* (outer) coating of bone. An excessive amount of pressure, such as lifting weights, can cause roughening of the ordinarily smooth *cartilagenous* surface of opposing bones.

40

A damaged joint can become the site of *traumatic arthritis*, which you recognize by the swelling from the build-up of mineral deposits and by chronically painful movement.

Once a joint exceeds its normal limit of movement and receives all or part of the damage listed above, it can become unstable—wobbly and unable to remain in its intended position, loose, weak and difficult to control when trying to support its ordinary weight-load.

THE MUSCLES

There are three types of muscle tissue in your body: *voluntary*, the muscles used to move bones, the "motor organs"; *involuntary*, the smooth muscle which cause movement in the glands, skin and organs—especially the stomach and intestines—and, *the heart muscle*, a special blend of fibers of both voluntary and involuntary types.

Muscles act like strings of the puppeteer, pulleys which move our limbs and spine in various directions. They have a broad attachment into the shaft or end of the bone they serve and, on the opposite end, insert into another bone which may be more fixed or less moveable.

Contracting muscle fibers pull the bone in a given direction. While this appears as a single movement, actually for every contraction there must be a simultaneous relaxation of the muscle with which it works—*synergistically*—in rhythmic harmony of contraction/relaxation.

Several muscle groups cooperate to permit you to raise your arm above your head. One group takes the arm to a

41

certain height, then releases while another group takes over. This process is repeated until eventually your arm is over your head. This relay effort—a series of simultaneous contractions and relaxations—is a classic example of *synergistic action.* Plainly the inability to move a part to its full expected limit may be caused by failure either to contract or relax in harmony.

Healthful muscle firmness is called "tone." A body out of shape, weak and unwilling to work, lacks sufficient "tone" to provide erectness of posture and the energy to accomplish ordinary work requirements of daily life. See Fig. 20.

LIGAMENTS

The Ligaments

Joints are held in place through ligaments, strong, semi-elastic *fibrous* bands composed of both *elastic* (yellow) and inelastic (white) fibers. An individual who can bend farther than average, like the so-called "double jointed" person, actually has more *yellow elastic* fibers in his or her ligaments than others, not a double joint.

In the spinal column there are two large, important ligaments concerned in backache. The *anterior* (front) *longitudental* ligament parallel to the spinal column. It does not cause pain.

The *posterior* (back) *longitudental* ligament which closely parallels the spine along the back is capable of producing pain. A disc or vertebra which is protruding

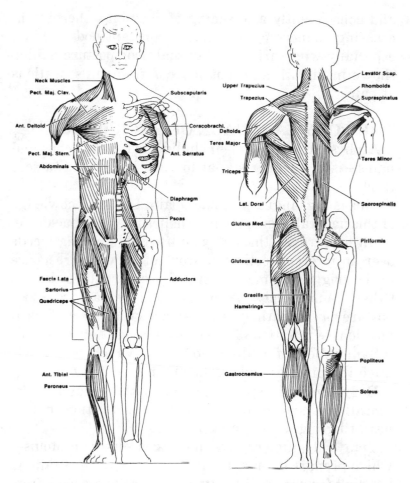

Fig. 20—Body muscles move harmoniously in all their actions.

and pushing backward against this ligament can cause constant sharp pain. Poor posture places a strain and a kink in the *posterior* ligament, especially when the spinal curves are exaggerated as in the cases of "sway back."

Aging is responsible for a loss of fluid in the ligaments,

and consequently a lessening of elasticity, thereby increasing chances for strain and constant body aching, especially when arising. Habitual poor posture habits, shown in Fig. 21, also contribute to frequent sensations of pain.

THE BODY LANGUAGE OF BACK PAIN

A physical symptom—including fearsome aches and pains—is a warning signal to your brain from a sore tissue.

This is the language of back pain. Use the knowledge of this natural phenomenon to help solve your backache.

An ache travels through your body at lightning speeds over an interconnecting network of nerves in response to the triggering mechanism of pressure upon tissues. Other causes may be mechanical imbalance—poor posture or repeating physical activities in awkward positions—irritation of noxious chemical substances or inflammation of a diseased organ which is reflexly affecting muscles and ligaments in your back.

Body language speaks to you in the vocabulary of sensations: heat, cold, pain, ache, constriction, numbness, tingling, boring and pressure.

Your body often receives messages—like symptoms—which prepare it for sudden movements, such as falling, bending forward and squatting. Injury to the neck from a rear-end collision occurs because your body is unprepared—thus unprotected—with the muscular contraction needed to withstand this impact. Receiving a blow without advance preparation sets the physical stage for the agony of whiplash.

You can strain your back merely by bending forward suddenly without prior muscular preparation.

44

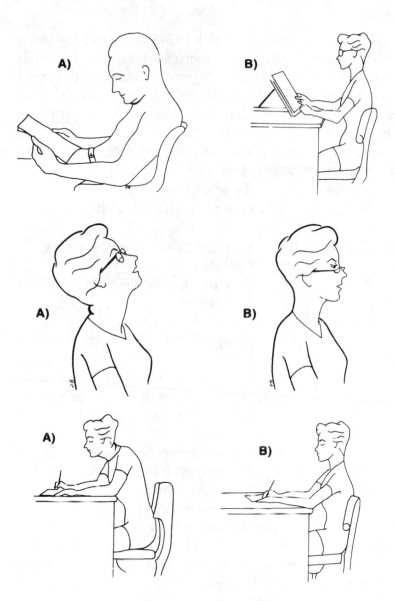

Fig. 21—Faulty habits (A) can be corrected (B) to prevent the neck pain and headache caused by repeated pressure on neck nerves.

Experiencing neck or back pain in either of the above circumstances is sufficient motive to learn how to decode the precise messages of body communication. It's to your advantage to interpret logically the signals sent by bone, muscle, ligament, tendon, nerve, blood vessel or through the pain referred by an organ.

Use the following chart to match the sensations to the corresponding anatomical chart:

Tissue	Type of Pain
Bone	Deep, knife-life, burning, stabbing
Muscle	Gripping, dull ache, throbbing, radiates
Nerve	Sharp, knife-like, shocking, radiates
Blood vessel	Burning, tingling, numbing, pressure pulsates with heart beat
Tendons	Pain associated with inflammation, constant dull ache, aggravated with body movement
Organs	Most are without pain fibers but do refer pain to muscles, frequently in the shoulder area.
Ligaments	Constant ache, bending movements aggravate

According to the literature, most organs are not equipped with pain fibers. However, the dull, boring pain of intestinal *colic* and an over-distended bladder appear to originate in the organ. It is believed the only adequate stimulus for organ pain is tension and distention of a hollow *viscus* (large organs of any one of the three cavities of the body).

ORGANS REFER PAIN TO THE BACK

If your major complaint is pain in the back, be alert to possible disease in an organ. A sick organ, such as the kidneys, liver, prostate, or ovaries, can refer pain to the back.

It makes good sense to realize a symptom of pain reflects your total state of health. Backache cannot be separated from your total being; it is just one aspect of your overall health.

Although this is a book about backache—not total health—it would be wise to examine yourself for all symptoms and signs of illness before starting your self-help program. If any doubt is raised by symptoms other than back pain, consider a professional consultation.

Although I believe anything can cause anything, and, maybe anything can cure anything, I also believe taking heavily advertised little liver pills which make you urinate is a long-shot to cure backache. It's just not the way to go.

A "reflex" nerve pathway carries pain from an inflamed organ to a distant part of the body by virtue of a "trigger" mechanism.

This is demonstrated in a person with an impacted kidney stone blocking the flow of urine to the bladder— a condition which "triggers" pain to the back, loins, groin and, in males, to the scrotum. Taking drugs which stimulate kidney activity and increase urine production is not advised.

Anyone who has felt back pain caused by a kidney stone will swear it is the most excruciating experience imaginable.

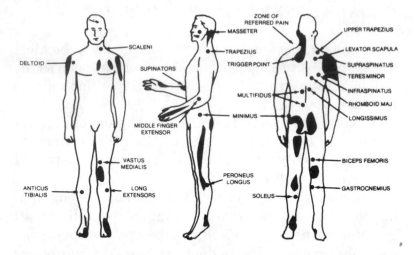

Fig. 22 illustrates the various trigger points, which when aggravated or irritated shoot sensations to other locations in the body. By testing the relative strength or weakness of the specific muscles listed in the drawings above, the doctor can determine the origin of the primary spinal disorder.

The stabbing sensation of a gall bladder "attack" has its champions, who claim this pain, which strikes beneath the shoulder blades, in the mid-spine and shoulder, is unbearable, second to none.

In females, a sagging *uterus* tugs on the ligamentous attachments in the back, causing low back pains, pressure sensations in the rectum, legs and thighs and distress in walking. A stretching of the *Fallopian tubes* produces some of these symptoms. A "kinked" *ureter* will cause nausea as well as other uncomfortable sensations, especially in response to jarring motions as in walking or other activities.

In males, the prostate gland refers pain into the rectum, lower back, groin and testicles. If this condition exists in conjunction with back strain in the lumbar region, intense pain is generated.

Chest pain is triggered by blockage of blood through the large or small arteries near the heart. Commonly this condition, known as *angina pectoris,* causes vice-like constriction of the chest, with extreme pain in the mid-spine area.

A rib misplaced from its attachment to a vertebra in

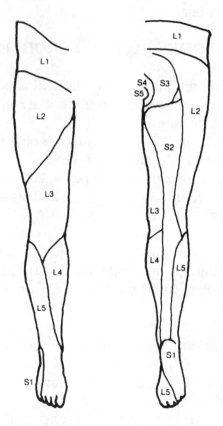

Fig. 23 shows the distribution of nerve flow from the lumbar and sacral nerves to the lower extremities. The sensations you experience in the legs may be originating in the lower back.

the back or sternum in front also will cause sharp chest pain which resembles heart trouble. However, rib pain differentiates itself from *angina* by being more localized to one specific spot.

In both men and women, malfunctions of sexual organs also affect the gastric functions, causing diarrhea, constipation, nausea and bloating. This general distress is associated with "pressure" sensations in the rectum, low back, and legs.

NEW ATTITUDES FOR OLD PROBLEMS

We've discussed many of the physical aspects of pain. Now let's focus on some of the emotional considerations, like general attitude.

This is an excellent time to adopt a new mental attitude toward your old back problems.

Learn to handle a painful experience productively.

When pain occurs, don't tense up and tighten all your body muscles into aching knots. RELAX YOURSELF.

Let yourself go limp. Take deep breaths and exhale slowly. Don't pant and allow the pain to consume your your total being. Do not hold your breath. This creates a negative pressure and heightens the pain, especially in the pelvic area.

When muscles become taut they compress and irritate the nerves which cause your pain. Cramping muscles can shut off the blood supply and cause more pain, primarily due to the congestion and swelling which occurs when blood cannot reenter the veinous return system. This syndrome activates chemical changes in glands which release substances into the bloodstream which further intensify the pain.

Tighten up and you're your own worst enemy. RELAX Let go.

Find a comfortable position (usually lying on the side opposite the pain with the knees drawn up to the chest in the fetal position) and, again, take long, slow measured breaths to reduce the blood pressure and pressure on the solar plexus and diaphragm.

Talk yourself into believing this pain will pass soon, and it will. Remember, if an individual can undergo surgery without anasthesia merely by autosuggestion (hypnosis), you can control this temporary moment of a painful episode.

This procedure follows a natural pathway by which you reverse negative learned responses.

You are now allowing the Central Nervous System (CNS) to behave in a more characteristic fashion by not prolonging pain with an overall response of distress.

Even a partial victory in this feedback experience is extremely rewarding. It has worked miracles for many cases of persistent backache and it's really not that difficult to accomplish if you put your mind to it. What you accomplish is a reversal of the destructive nervous patterns established through fear of what was happening to your body.

Having the knowledge and understanding of your problem helps free you from the bondage of fear and pain, the byproduct of your past fear, subsequent tension and stress.

Nerves become deadened after prolonged stimulation. Take advantage of this. Keep a constructive, positive attitude. Believe that pain has subsided, even though this may be a reversal of your customary attitude. A new mental image of your condition will help work a change for the good. Practice it!

Remember that your health is *your* responsibility, not that of your doctor. He is responsible for guiding you, for providing information to help restore you to normal, but the rest is up to you.

Follow his instructions. Take command. Generate enthusiasm and positivism to overcome your health problems.

To accomplish this, you must have faith in your doctor. If this is lacking, the chances of recovery and enthusiasm to get well will arrive slowly, if at all.

WHAT A GOOD DOCTOR CAN DO FOR YOU

Every person expects different things from his or her doctor. It's in an emergency situation that our priority is highest. We truly believe survival is impossible without the highest quality of professional care to repair the broken bones and mend the cut, torn and mangled tissues and organs. We want our lives saved.

Any disagreement here?

On the other hand, should you expect less from the person you visit for back pain? Many people do, and it's important that you not be one of them.

A good doctor for you is one skilled in back problems. Regardless of what "kind" of doctor, he must understand how to locate your problem and relieve it.

A bad doctor is one who is not skilled or thorough in his examination process, he skips over much of the vital information. He may feel that backs are not his thing.

Take the case of the young intern on his first house call, who studied the woman patient for so long that she asked, "What's wrong with me, doc?"

"I don't know . . . but, I sure wish you were pregnant . . . I'm a whiz at delivering babies."

Without knowing what's wrong, there's only a slim chance of fixing it, as my patient, Mrs. Bromley discovered.

A forty-five year old businesswoman, Mrs. Bromley was very abrupt in her manner. Although referred to me by another patient, she was obviously skeptical.

"Why are you making me bend in all these directions?"

"Didn't your other doctor make you do this?" I asked.

"No, he didn't. And, why are feeling my naked back?"

"I'm looking for muscle spasms and possible malalignments of the vertebra."

"My other doctor didn't do that," she said. "Actually, I wondered how he could know what was wrong with my back without touching it. But, I just felt he knew what he was doing and I shouldn't question him."

Mrs. Bromley's case ended more pleasantly than it began. Now she can spend the whole day on her feet without a sharp, stabbing pain in the low back.

Her problem was located and corrected by removing the source of irritation in the lower vertebra. She referred her sister to me and rather than questions, the sister made an initial demand: "I want you to feel my back—right here—just like you did to my sister. I know this is where my problem is."

And it was! All family members deserve skilled care.

Charles Bonnett, M.D., a specialist in spinal curvature (scoliosis) treatment believes, "Family doctors generally practice medicine only on their patient's front half, especially when they are examining children."

As Chief of the spinal deformity service at Rancho Los Amigos in Los Angeles, Dr. Bonnett says, "Scoliosis is

53

not merely a matter of appearance, it is associated with the premature development of osteoarthritis and severe cases can lead to early death from heart failure."

Parents who have back conditions should consider examinations for their children, as well as themselves.

"Parents should check their children's spines by closely examining them in the nude during their growing years," says Dr. Walter P. Blount, Milwaukee's world renowned authority on deformities of the spine. "Even small curves should be treated."

Arnold Fox, M.D., a director of the American Institute of Health, brings to focus the attitude of health with his message of "The New Health" found in *Let's Live* Magazine.

"The key to The New Health is to first learn about yourself, Don't rely solely on your doctor to tell you what he thinks is wrong with your body, what nutrients your system needs, how various substances harm your body, and how stress affects you and how to deal with it."

More about forming a satisfactory doctor/patient relationship will be found in Chapter 6.

RELIEF IS NOT FOUND IN A LABEL

A single term will not always describe an abnormal condition. Usually, as with many cases of back pain, there are many causes and many symptoms.

Consider the common cold, the label covering a group of symptoms—fever, muscle aching, headache, runny nose, lung congestion, throat inflammation and eliminative upset and general fatigue.

Would calling a cold *Rhinitis*, meaning inflammation of the mucous membranes of the nose, alter its course of recovery? Hardly.

A technical label—*a diagnosis*—will not cure backache either. Of course, descriptive terms are necessary for communication. But, *diagnosis* does not convey a cure.

I want my patients to know as much about their problem as I can. Every person, I believe, has the right to share knowledge about his or her body with the attending doctor. This is my obligation under the implied contract of a doctor/patient relationship. It is also the practice ethic of the chiropractic profession.

Despite best efforts at all times, I experience an occassional failure through my fault, that of my assistants or due to a patient not carrying out orders.

One of my less-than-perfect cases was Agnes, a likable, unmarried, middle-aged electronics assembler. She wasn't satisfied with my assessment of her injuries, resulting from rolling over in her Volkswagen.

To justify her contention, she traveled to the Mayo Clinic, to the Osteopathic Hospital in Kirksville, MO. and, finally, to the Stanford Memorial Hospital, Palo Alto, CA where she received a complete neurological examination. Each institution summed up its examination findings of her injuries with the identical phrase: "Soft tissue damage associated with cervical strain/ sprain," which was the original diagnosis I had made.

The treatment prescribed by each clinic was Darvon and Valium.

Agnes learned that what you call an ailment doesn't make it well. She paid dearly to learn this simple bit of logic because, now she could be a victim of drug dependency.

The mutiple causes of backache may generate a bombardment of symptoms.

A primary muscle cramp constricts the blood vessels which, in turn, respond with throbbing and sensations of pressure, commonly in the rectal area. Straining at stool, coughing, sneezing or laughing causes symptoms of pressure in the pelvic area and legs. Irritating or stretching a nerve causes a radiation of pain to surrounding or distant areas which are interconnected with the nerve pathway (Fig. X). Digestive and sexual organs are stimulated or deadened by a change in flow of the endocrine glands. Arthritic deposits accumulate at joints when liver, spleen or kidney functions are disturbed. Stiffness occurs in joints when the ligaments lose their fluid content and elasticity, mainly due to over-stretching, nutritional abuse and aging.

While locating the source of your back pain is the first—and most significant—procedure to end backache, many patients are subjected to the expense of over-examination, and unnecessary diagnostic procedures.

A recent article in the magazine "RN"—a journal for registered nurses and students—reported a poll of 12,500 nurses revealed they "no longer take a physician's word for granted . . . nor should the patient be expected to."

"The number of unnecessary procedures conducted every day," was one of the determining factors in the nurses' attitude to lean in favor of the patient, rather than blindly follow hospital policies and orders of doctors which disregard considerations affecting the patient's welfare.

Marvin S. Belsky, M.D., and Leonard Gross have coauthored *Beyond The Medical Mystique—How To Choose Your Doctor* (Priam Books, New York)—if you want additional reference on this interesting subject.

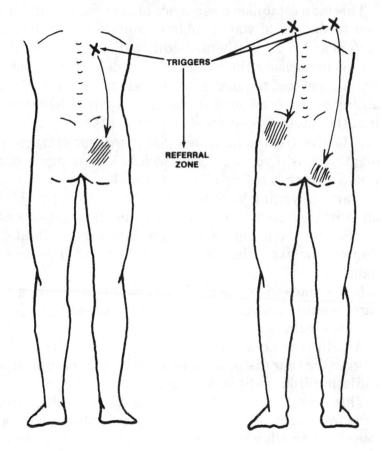

Fig. X demonstrates the areas of pain referred from upper levels of the lumbar or thoracic spinal regions. When the sciatic nerve is involved, pain may extend all the way to the foot and toes. Pain may be triggered by a muscle spasm, pressure on a nerve root or by alteration in blood supply to the area.

THE STEPS TO DISCOVERY

Following in the centuries-old footsteps of health practitioners will lead you to a solution of your backache.

This is an established sequence of events which guides you to the site of your problem, isolates the irratative factors and removes them. Additionally, it provides the means to measure the extent of your defect—the shortness of one leg, the degree of spinal curve, the limited ability to perform certain physical activities like bending, the intensity and frequency of distress.

Effective treatment allows you to measure improvement, just as if you were on a weight loss program you would expect to see results on the scale.

Start by writing your medical history. This provides an intimate insight into your overall health behavior and it rules out the presence of major pathology or disease. Cancer, for example, also causes back and hip-socket pain.

Make notes to yourself of prior accident, injuries or significant illnesses. List all of your symptoms, not just the back pain.

An allied or associated problem could actually be the trigger for your discomfort, especially in the case of pain radiating from a diseased organ.

This procedure will bring remarkable results, even in cases where others have told you "nothing can be done." After all, who is more familiar with your body than you are?

Remember, consult a professional if you uncover facts which alarm you.

"If you don't know what's wrong with it, how in the world are you ever going to fix it?" My mother used this expression frequently. Does its simplistic logic falter when applied to your health?

When acute back pain propels you into the doctor's office, do you wonder if anyone will know enough about your problem to fix it? And, following a brief examination, are you puzzled how the examiner found out so much about you so swiftly? Are you bewildered that anyone can sort through all the anatomical parts of your wonderful body and reach a conclusion?

You are about to find out how.

CHAPTER 3
How To Find Clues
To Your Condition

When asked by Dr. Watson how he had solved a puzzling crime, Sherlock Holmes would usually reply, "By deduction, my dear Watson, by deduction."

A crime of sorts is being committed by your body against your body or else you wouldn't have a backache. By using deduction like Holmes—better yet, detailed investigation—you may be able to solve it—to find the offender.

You start with observation.

How do key parts of your body look while performing certain revealing physical movements?

It's not always easy to appraise yourself objectively during such maneuvers, so you want the help of a doctor or a relative or friend.

However, you go ahead with your self-evaluation, check the way you move. Are you smooth, well-balanced or uncoordinated, out of rhythm and jerky?

Here are points to check.

See if one leg or foot appears to drag, turn in or outward, or if one hip or shoulder is high, as if you're heading north and south at the same time.

If your belly-button—known in learned circles as *umbilicus*—points away from the center line—left or right—and your torso is twisted, you have a pelvic rotation or twisted hip. Any observer can easily note this defect while you walk.

As you move through each step of the self-evaluation, try to decide if the defect found is the primary cause of your problem—or if it is a secondary or compensatory abnormality.

Remember the integrity of your whole body depends on the proper alignment and working of each part.

Everything you find wrong must be corrected ... the posture, spinal curves, muscle weakness, for example, before mechanical balance can be restored to the body's entire frame.

Sometimes it is possible to correct the primary cause only. The secondary—compensation—effects disappear of their own accord.

A side-view of your erect stance reveals the state of your posture. Compare the way you stand to the posture model illustrated in Fig. 6.

Are the curves in the neck, mid-back and low back within normal range? Determine if a plumb-line would fall from the ear, through the shoulder, midway through the chest, hip and knee and end at the ankle, like the model's.

(If you find gross postural differences from the "normal," you'll benefit from the Perfect Posture Chart. Merely by looking, and comparing yourself to the model—every day—will speed your return to the healthy erectness which brings relief from muscular tension, stress and pain.)

For the extra deep curve in the lower back, practice the exercises shown in Fig. 24 for correction of "sway back" (lumbar lordosis) caused by a forward-drooping pelvis.

Correct shoulders which droop downward and forward causing a lump or hump in the mid-back by standing with the back flat against a wall. Elevate the chest, feeling the muscular contraction in the stomach area,

61

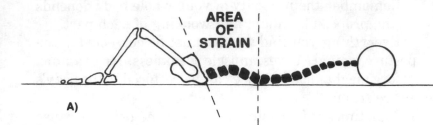

A)

AREA OF STRAIN

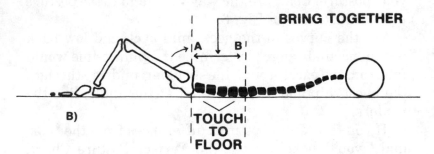

B)

BRING TOGETHER

A ← → B

TOUCH TO FLOOR

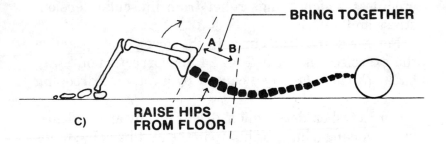

C)

BRING TOGETHER

A → B

RAISE HIPS FROM FLOOR

Fig. 24—Getting rid of the pain of "sway" back the permanent way. This is undoubtedly the most common of all postural faults responsible for backache. The effects of this bad habit can be overcome by practicing the following exercise ten to fifteen minutes daily. You will strengthen weak abdominal and buttock muscles which allow the pelvis to fall forward, the undesirable action which puts a "sway" (lumbar lordosis) in your lower spine. Lie on the floor with a pillow under your head to prevent neck strain. Visualize your lower back being glued to the floor. When you have mastered this exercise lying down, practice standing and sitting with the buttocks "tucked" under.
A) This is your trouble area. See how the angle of the pelvis is increased when the low back curve is increased, causing strain on back muscles and ligaments. It also causes pressure on the disc separating the last vertebra (fifth) with the sacrum and the spinal nerve. The normal angle is shown in Fig. B.
B) Lying on the floor, pull upward from the pelvis (pubes) by contracting the buttock and abdominal muscles in harmony. Pull point A and point B together. Keep the back flat.
C) When step B becomes easily performed, advance to step C. Raise your entire lower back upward from the surface as shown. Keep points A and B squeezed together. Raise and lower repeatedly.

site of the *solar plexus* and *diaphragm.*

Be certain the ear—and the head—is directly above the shoulder. If the ear is forward of the shoulder, this head action pulls the shoulders forward—and downward—allowing the shoulders to droop. This attitude further depresses the chest, lowering the vital holding capacity of the lungs. When you are unable to fill the lungs and draw in a full measure of air you are creating "tiredness" due to lack of oxygen intake. Also, because this makes the heart beat faster to supply tissues with adequate amounts of blood, you encourage high blood pressure.

You can correct the habit of a "forward head carriage" by standing with your back flat against a wall. Draw your chin backward—look straight ahead, not up—without raising your chin. Tuck your chin into the neck, rather than allowing it to point upward.

Use caution not to point your chin upward. This common, bad, and costly habit puts an undesirable super-curve in your neck, causing destructive pressure on the cervical discs. Habitually bending the head upward (raising the chin) is due to eye strain, poor vision, use of poorly made bifocals, or, simply the result of an acquired postural habit (Fig. 17). The sooner you break this habit, the quicker you'll experience relief from muscular problems in this area of the back.

If you're shorter than average, overcome the tendency to look up at the person you're talking to. Instead, take one step backward and aim your eyeballs upward to the other person. This simple practice will add years to the pain-free function of neck tissues.

The next step in your evaluation is movement. This will reveal the exact spot of your pain.

For a hip problem, for example, bend in each direction and stop at the exact instant—and position—pain occurs. You may have to bend, squat, stoop or twist to re-duplicate the action or position which triggers your pain.

Once it's found, you'll have a target to reach with the corrective exercises found in the last chapter. You'll know where help is needed to end your backache, and which specific exercises will relieve your problem.

So far you've made only a topographical excursion of your body. It doesn't account for internal factors—body chemistry, glandular or digestive functions or the results of your conscious and subconscious emotional output upon the musculo-skeletal structures.

Don't be overly concerned with these secondary aspects at this point. The Art of Healing is covered in Chapter 5. Right now you're prepared to find additional clues of your imbalance which will be revealed by the various tissues and anatomical parts of your body.

Since the lower half of the body is most commonly affected with backache, start your examination here. You should be naked, or wear brief underclothing to provide full inspection.

THE WALK (GAIT)

As a trained observer, I know how revealing walking can be. It opens a window to an individual's working machinery. It instantly discloses many things about a person's condition, including some diseases ranging from brain damage to syphillis. So, don't fail to walk back and forth several times for your observer. Allow for an inventory of all existing imperfections.

The walk *(gait)* (Fig. 25) shows action in the feet, legs and body and the existing relationship of these independent parts to the whole body in the act of motion. called *kinetic behavior* (Fig. 26).

Both legs should move equally in speed and distance with a harmonious action. Both knees should rise equally in height. The foot should strike the floor on the heel with a forward, rolling motion on the entire foot (Fig. 27). the lift-off should be even, not on the inner or outer foot surface (Fig. 28). See if a foot points (toes) in or out. Body imbalance is first detected when one or both ankles bend inward or outward while standing or walking (observed best from the rearview while standing with both feet together) (Fig. 9).

The arms should swing freely and equally in a criss-cross action with legs. The left arm, for example, should swing forward with the right leg. If this is not occur-

65

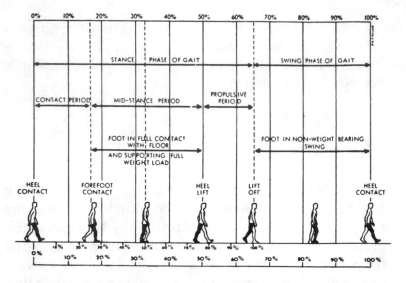

Fig. 25—The walking gait.

ring, problems affecting body coordination will occur. Correct this by crawling on the floor five minutes each day for two weeks, then recheck your walk. It could be normal now. If not, wait two weeks and repeat the process.

(In the motion picture "North Dallas Forty" recall how Robert Preston—my old classmate—crawled on the floor with Burt Reynolds?)

If your head is tilted to one side, use that standard exercise of schools for models, practice walking with a book balanced on your head to correct this bad postural habit, which is responsible for neck, shoulder and back tension, eye-strain and headache.

The knees should not bend backward unnecessarily—in fact, there should be a slight forward *(flexion)* knee bend—when walking. If the knee is in this former position *(hyper-extension)*, it is possible to change the center

66

KINETIC STANCE PHASE OF GAIT

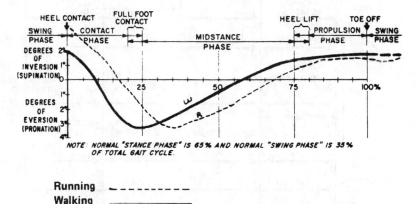

NOTE: NORMAL "STANCE PHASE" IS 65% AND NORMAL "SWING PHASE" IS 35% OF TOTAL GAIT CYCLE.

Running   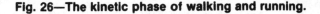
Walking

Fig. 26—The kinetic phase of walking and running.

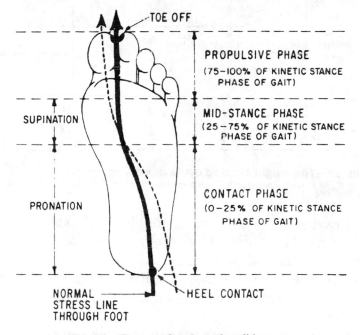

Fig. 27—The mechanics of walking.

67

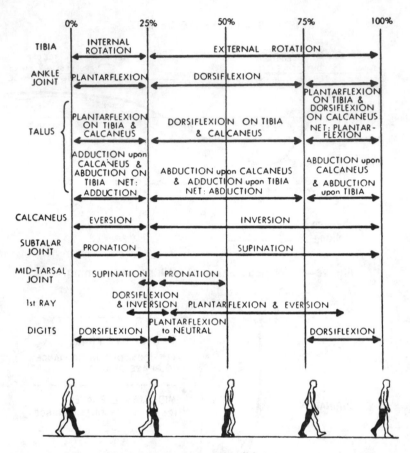

Fig. 28—The weight bearing cycle of walking.
(Figs. 25, 26, 27 and 28 courtesy of The Foot Book, Harry F. Hlavic, M. Ed., D.P.M., World Publishing, Mt. View, CA).

of gravity by raising the normal level of axis (Fig. 29). The knee is required to rise abnormally to counteract this gravitational imbalance.

Running—and runners—requires excellent posture to avoid structural damage, such a strain, to the feet. legs and back.

The average person's step is 25-inches long, and he

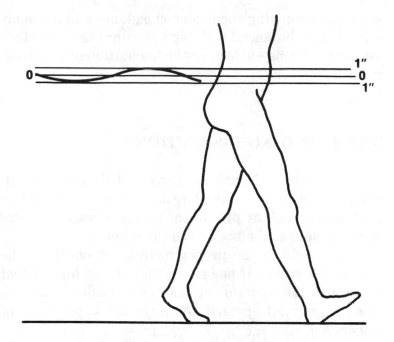

Fig. 29—The axis of your center of gravity fluctuates approximately 2″ during movement of walking. Bending the knees too far backward (hyperextension) can alter the normal rhythmic flow in the pelvic area.

takes about 90 to 120 steps per minute.

Gait push-off may be affected by arthritis or a painful condition in the great toe. Another cause for a lop-sided push-off may be weakness in the muscles of the buttocks *(gluteus maximus)* or calves *(gastrocnemius, soleus* and *flexor hallucis longus)*. A lurch during the midstance may involve weakness in the *gluteus medius* muscle. (Consult the diagram of body muscles).

Unusual gait is commonly and frequently associated with weak muscles of the buttocks and legs. Since the action of walking is controlled through these muscle groups, it is important to determine which muscle group

69

is weak, permitting the incorrect cadence and harmony required for balanced walking and running—and other *kinetic* functions—affecting the foundation of the structural framework.

THE STANDING INSPECTION

Check front and back for abnormal signs of inflammation, swelling, discoloration, and asymetrical landmarks, such as prominent lumps or valleys. Compare one side of the body with the other.

(Fig. 30) shows the proper method for checking the level of the pelvis. If one side is higher, the hip is tilted or rotated. Rotation pulls the leg on the side of the high *ilium* (hip bone) upward and gives the appearance of a short leg.

The hip may become twisted—rotated—due to strain in the lumbar muscles, a lateral spinal curvature, or an immovable fixation in the several movable joints located here: The ball and socket joint of the hip proper and the pelvic joints, the *ilium, sacrum,* and *fifth lumbar vertebra,* see Fig. 1.

From the back, see if the skin folds defining the lower level of the buttock are level, (Fig. 31). A tilted pelvis allows one hip to drop.

Find the two buttock dimples located close to the tailbone. These, also, will show the level of the pelvis, similarly to the buttock skin folds.

Two simple tests will reveal a hip problem.

The Trendelenburg test is positive, indicating a problem, if the buttock drops lower than the opposite when

70

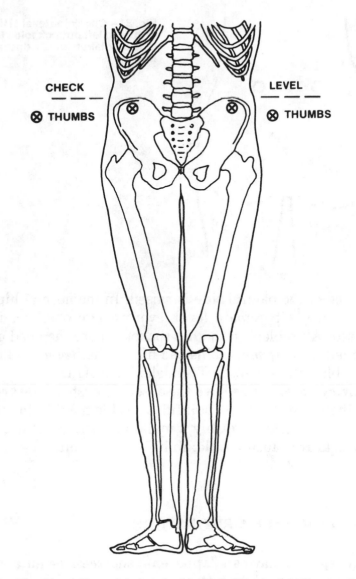

Fig. 30—Check the pelvis by placing both thumbs into the small depression found near the top of the large bones in the hip. If one thumb is higher than the other, the pelvis is tilted or rotated upward and backward.

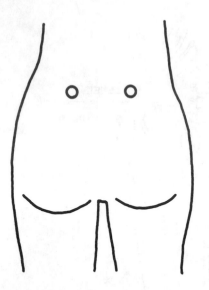

Fig. 31—Check the level of the right and left buttock folds for pelvic rotation or an uneven hip.

the leg of the painful side is raised. In the normal hip, both sides will remain level, even though one knee is raised. A problem in the hip socket, where the head of the leg bone, *(femur)* joins the hip at the *ilium*, also is possible with a positive Trendelenburg sign.

Lying on your side have the observer push downward on the ilium. If this is painful, a problem exists in the *sacro-iliac* joint, probably a malalignment or arthritic deposits are causing inflexibility in this joint.

TESTING FOR A SHORT LEG

A leg may have an "apparent" shortness or an anatomical—real—shortness.

One leg can be shorter—an anatomical shortness—due to injury, disease or a congenital defect, failure in natural bone development.

A leg can also have an "apparent" shortness, especially on weightbearing, due to rotation of the hip, muscle and ligament strain, or imbalanced muscles—either weakness or *spasm (involuntary contraction)*—on opposite sides of the body.

Check for an apparent shortness by measuring from the belly button *(umbilicus)* to the small bump on the inner surface of the ankle, the *medial* (middle) *malleolus* (Fig. 32, A and B).

A short leg can be responsible for continual body imbalance. It will produce annoying problems from foot to head. A headache, for example, may clear when legs are evened, and the entire body is rebalanced. Your doctor may make the adjustment necessary to level the pelvis. Additionally, he may suggest building up one shoe or adding a lift to the heel to overcome unyielding causes for a short leg.

When a short leg is found, you can determine which bone of the leg is affected, the *femur* or the *tibia*, see Fig. 34.

Irregularity in the hip level causes formation of a lateral (sideways) curve in the low back.

Nature compensates for this cure by causing an offsetting curve to form in the mid-back, a secondary curve. Ordinarily, correcting the primary low back curve will cause the secondary, mid-back, curve to disappear.

REFERRED PAIN

Pain may be referred to the hip from the knee as well as from the lower *(lumbar)* spine, as shown in Fig. 35.

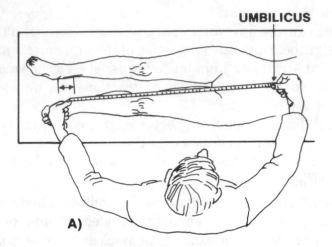

UMBILICUS

A)

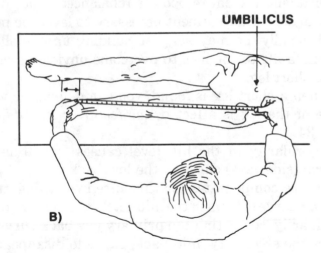

UMBILICUS

B)

Fig. 32—Method of checking for a "short" leg. A) An apparent shortness in one leg may be due to muscle tightness, rotation in the pelvis
and lumbar vertebral malalignment. B) A true short leg is the result of
an abnormalacy, fracture or other deficit in normal growth and development. A true short leg measures the same whether standing or
lying. Both conditions warrant treatment to correct the body imbalance.

74

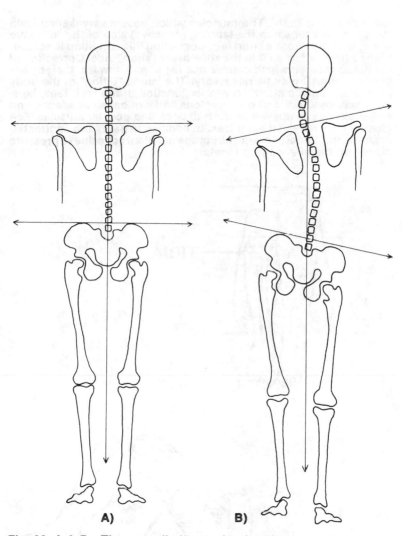

A)   B)

Fig. 33, A & B—The over-all effects of a short leg are easily seen by comparing figure A with Figure B. This deficiency is related to physical problems occuring from the feet to the head. It causes displacement of organs as well as the structures which support your body in an upright position against the gravitational pull. Unless the exercises you practice are designed specifically for correction of the specific muscle groups made weak by this imbalance, you could be further

75

damaging your body. The muscles which become weakened from imbalance are those on the leaning (concave) side of the "c" curve which develops from a short leg. Correcting this condition is accomplished by wearing a lift in the shoe of the "short" side. Correction of the pelvic rotation which causes one leg to pull upward, thereby becoming "short," may be necessary. The lateral "tilting" of the body generates complications on proper function in the feet, legs, hips, low back, shoulder and neck regions and can cause headache and eye strain due to uneven tension of neck and occular muscles. See chapter 8 for remedial exercises. In addition to pain from contracted muscles, this condition will encourage constant ache due to pressure placed on the interlocking facets.

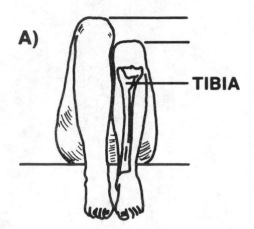

A)

TIBIA

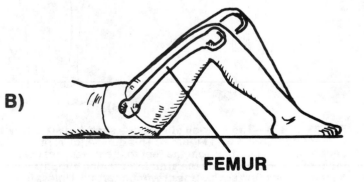

B)

FEMUR

Fig. 34—Method to determine if leg shortness occurs in A) the Tibia or B) the Femur bone.

76

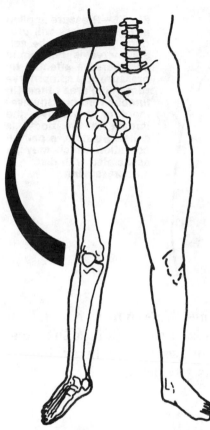

Fig. 35—Shows how pain may be referred to the hip from both the knee and lower back.

Sciatica—inflammation of the *sciatic* nerve—results from exceptional pressure on the nerve emitting between the lower *lumbar vertebra*. Extreme pain starts in the low back and extends into the buttocks and down the back of the leg, ending slightly above the knee.

Fig. 36 shows the location in the buttock of the sciatic nerve. Slight pressure over this point will produce pain if the sciatic nerve is involved and inflamed.

A pain similar to that of sciatica is caused by rupture (herniation) of an intervertebral disc, the elastic pad-

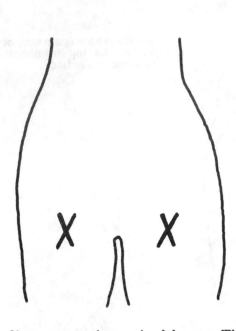

Fig. 36—Pressure applied at the "X" mark will produce pain when the sciatic nerve is inflammed or otherwise affected by pressure on a spinal nerve root in the area of the 4th lumbar vertebra. Involvement of this nerve, the largest in the body, is called Sciatica, a painful condition which may be associated with disc embarassment.

ding separating spinal bones. This, however, is felt in the groin and down the back of the leg to the little toe.

If your low back pain follows this pathway, have a professional consultation as soon as possible.

TESTING FOR MUSCLE STRENGTH

While the obvious emphasis is on muscles of the back—prime offenders in a backache—equal focus must be made on the front muscles, those in the abdomen.

Clearly. vertical balance must engage the muscles of both the front *and* back of the erect body. Frequently, problems of poor posture—and subsequent backache—originate in weak abdominal muscles which fail to carry their load in maintaining equilibrium.

78

Here's how to tell if inadequate abdominal strength is the culprit in your back pain.

Lie on your back with feet together and pull upward, as shown in Fig. 37. If your low back rises off the table, "C," abdominal muscles are weak. Furthermore, you have an anterior tilt to the pelvis and both these factors are causing serious and constant low back strain. Check yourself for excessive curve in the low back ("sway back").

STRENGTHENING ABDOMINAL MUSCLES

Three easy movements will strengthen the lower and upper abdominal muscles.

1. Try this exercise five minutes daily for the lower abdominals: Lie on the back with a rolled towel or small pillow under the knees. Put your hands beside your head and flatten the back to the floor or table by pulling upward from the *pubes*, where the two pelvic bones come together in the front, see Fig. 24. Contract the abdominal muscles. By taking easy, full breaths, you relax the "upper" abdominal muscles, which is necessary for proper action. Remember, don't allow the low back to arch or come up off the table.

2. This exercise is performed in the same position. However, instead of having both feet together, allow one heel to glide headward, toward your buttock. Now, pull the other bent leg toward the buttocks. Return each leg the same way. Again, keep the back flat against the table. If the low back arches, start the exercise over, you are not doing it correctly.

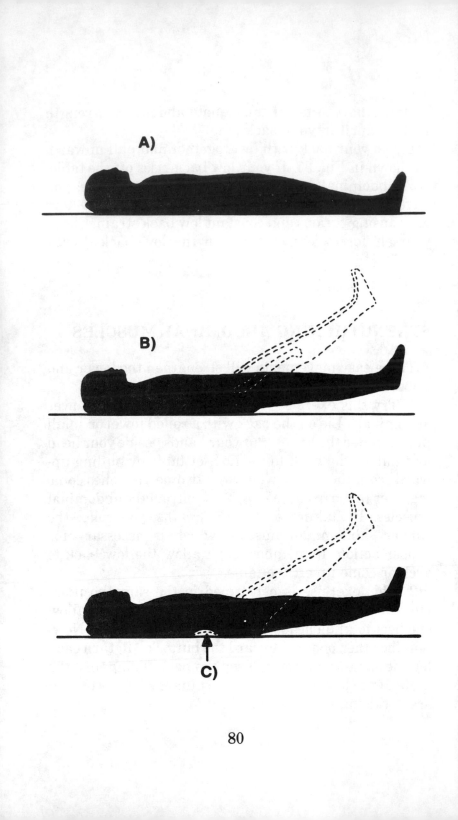

Fig. 37—Movements involved in double leg-raising. A) the first phase shows a posterior tilting of the pelvis done by the abdominal muscles. B) this individual is strong enough to hold the pelvis in a posterior tilt throughout the whole movement. C) the pelvis is in a position of anterior tilt, which occurs with insufficient strength to prevent the weight of the legs from tilting the pelvis forward. The dotted line shows how, when the legs are raised, the back curve tends to decrease.

3. To strengthen the "upper" abdominals, pull about 8 inches off the table from a lying flat position with arms extended, see Fig. 38. Do not exceed eight inches, and do not allow anyone to hold your feet. Again, try to hold the low back flat to the table (A), because this area, along with the abdominal muscles, is what the exercises are aiming to correct.

Avoid "push-ups" or raising and holding the feet in the air while lying flat. These exercises are contraindicated where weakness exists in abdominal muscles.

TESTING FOR RANGE-OF-MOVEMENT

Warning! Proceed with caution if you don't know the range-of-motion of your body joints!

You can get into serious trouble.

Here's a good way to test to see if any or many of your muscle groups are not flexible enough. Just imitate the action in the following illustrations.

81

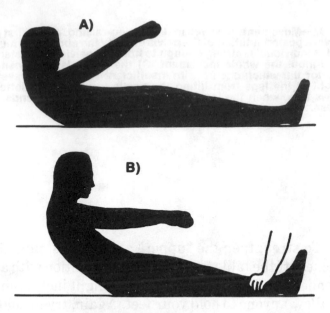

Fig. 38—In A) the action is chiefly trunk flexion . . .raising the upper trunk and tilting the pelvis backward. You are using the abdominal muscles. In B) the position of trunk flexion is held by the abdominal muscles while the movement is flexion of the pelvis on the thighs, performed by the hip flexor muscles.

It's easy to experience muscle and ligament strain in an area of restricted motion. Your brain sometimes moves faster than your body. It's impossible to remember exactly how far you can—and can't—move. Therefore, a sudden impulse causes a swift bending action, and, ouch!—there's a pain, and possibly work or play time lost, because you're flat on your back.

A simple solution is to find your area of muscle tightness, as demonstrated with the illustrations, Fig. 39, A to G. Do the specific exercises which loosen tight muscles, and restrict movement. And as a pre-cautionary mea-

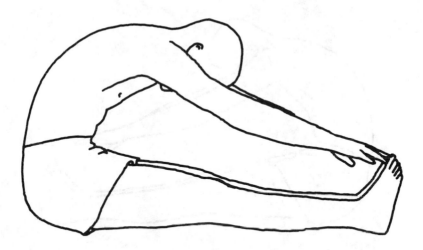

Fig. 39—This shows the normal bending action of the trunk. Compare how closely you resemble this drawing.

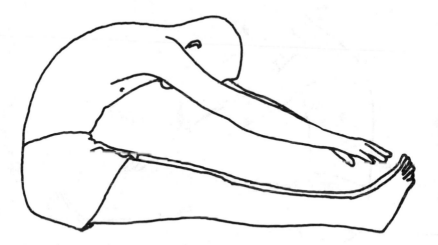

Fig. 39-A—While the back is bending adequately, it is impossible to bend the toes upward, indicating tightness in the calf muscles.

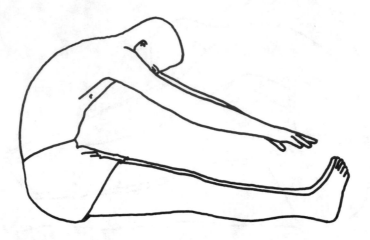

Fig. 39-B—The failure to touch the toes is due to tightness in the rear thigh muscles *(hamstrings).*

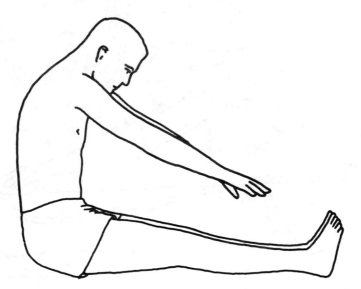

Fig. 39-C—The obvious tightness here in the lower back muscles.

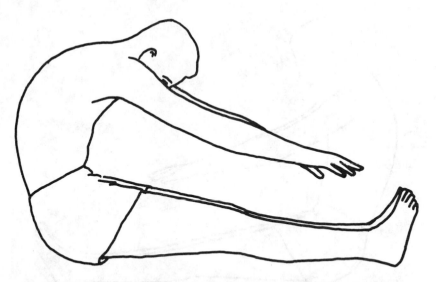

Fig. 39-D—While it appears this subject is bending far, the movement is mainly in the upper back, which could be excessively loose, or slack, while the tightness is shown by lack of bending in the low back and slight raising of the knees to tightness in back of the thighs, *(the hamstrings)*.

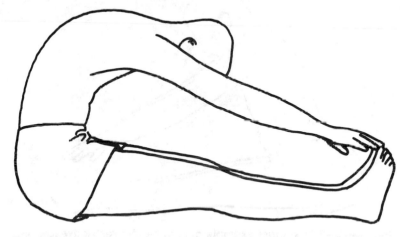

Fig. 39-E—This is an exaggeration of the previous example   of slackness in the upper spine associated with tightness in the low back and stretched *hamstrings*.

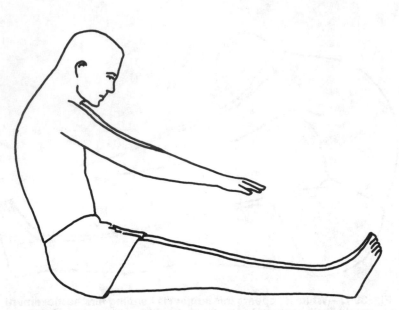

Fig. 39-F—This is an example of an extreme tightness in muscles of the low back, hamstrings, and calf muscles.

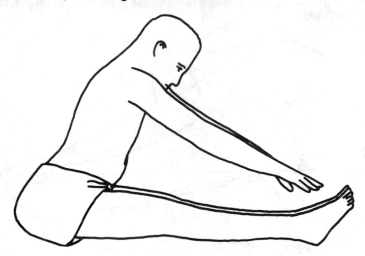

Fig. 39-G—Still another example of super-tight, restrictive low back muscles. The upper back muscles are of normal length.

sure, remember to avoid sudden moves, like forward bending, without first preparing the body.

Let me remind you that proper joint movement is the result of both muscle contraction and relaxation. Also, remember that weakness, rather than strength, is the worst offender in limiting range of motion.

Now that you have some ideas about your limitations, you are about to gain insights to the nervous system— which controls the sensations and triggers many of the muscular responses. This will lead you another step closer to your goal of getting rid of the cause of your back pain.

CHAPTER 4
Unlock The Mysteries Of
The Nervous System

This chapter could be eliminated *if* there was a way to spare you from unraveling the "mystery" of the nervous system—how it works to rack your body with pain, and how you can control it to end a siege of backache.

A clue to the overall significance of the nervous system is contained in this statement from *Brain and Mind*, by R.J. Berry, M.D.

"There can be no disease which does not disturb the nerve cells concerned; hence it is important for these conducting nerve pathways to be studied from the modern standpoint of the ingoing or *receptor nerve impulses* and the outgoing or *effector* ones. If the cause of the disturbance of these conducting nerves can be ascertained or removed, the patient will be cured. If not, treatment merely diverts attention from the truth."

My experience with Jerry, a 38-year-old, high-rise steel worker, sharply illustrates the problems of misunderstanding the nervous system.

Jerry was in agony, the result of a low back pain. His back muscles resembled the steel cables supporting the Golden Gate Bridge, where he worked.

"What the hell's wrong with my back? *This pain!* I can't stand it." Jerry wasn't kidding. "I'll jump off the bridge if you can't help me!"

That shook me up. Holding constant pressure on various pain-points, I made slight adjustments in the low spine, and Jerry relaxed a bit, experiencing enough relief to go home. I was more than a little concerned when he failed to return the next day as instructed.

Two days later he reappeared, looking and smelling like something from the gutter, his worried wife in his wake.

"What's happened, Jerry?"

"He's been drunk for two days," his wife explained.

"But why?" I asked.

"To deaden his nerves so he wouldn't feel the pain."

Then it dawned on me that Jerry had probably followed this drastic—and wrong—course because he had taken literally the common expression characterizing drunkenness—"feeling no pain."

Drinking had brought about the opposite result—extreme rectal pain. Quickly I relieved Jerry's agony by applying a cold-pack to the low back, explaining that alcohol had not deadened his nerves. It had actually inflamed them, adding the pain from his rectum to that of his back.

"How big is a nerve?" Jerry wanted to know.

"Anywhere between the thickness of a hair to that of the lead in a pencil. However, the sciatic nerve, which is giving you fits in the buttock and leg, can be swollen to the size of your thumb."

"How can anything that little hurt so much?" Jerry asked.

Jerry stayed sober and in time quit hurting. He also learned that inside one "nerve"—even the size of the lead in a pencil—are hundreds of individual fibers which may make four-hundred interconnections with muscles and other nerves.

A back pain is not the fault of just one isolated tiny-sized nerve; it involves the entire nervous system, which connects everything in the body to everything, figuratively speaking.

If you imagine billions upon billions of cells housed with the skull—the home of your central nervous system—you can sense how vast is your body's communicating network.

The central nervous system (CNS) receives data from your external environment, and relates this to your internal environment, the living world inside you, establishing equilibrium within your body.

The brain is a miraculous communication center. Neither IBM computer technology nor Ma Bell's wizardry will ever duplicate the workability or sophistication of this engineering masterpiece.

It's difficult to imagine all the different functions of the body constantly being monitored by the brain—like an intergalactic traffic cop, keeping the millions of stars and moons in their proper places.

Signals speed like rockets back and forth between the brain and your body as you read this page:

Nerves to the brain control the muscles of your eyes and pupils, causing the eyeball to follow the printed words and the pupils to dilate to allow more light, in addition to controlling focus to lenses of the eyes to enable you to read. Muscles contract and relax to maintain your reading position comfortably, without effort or thought. Body temperature is regulated, causing you to sweat if too warm, or shiver if too cold. Food within your stomach is digested, and after being absorbed and assimilated within the small intestine will enter the bloodstream, providing energy to keep you reading.

The liver and kidneys are filtering out specific chemicals, delivering them to the proper location for storage or elimination. The heart keeps pumping 76 times per minute, while blood pressure is maintained at 120/80. All this time you are taking a measured 16 breaths per minute while exchanging carbon dioxide from the lungs with the inflow of oxygen-containing fresh air.

It's a fabulous scenario. From inception in the womb to your last breath, all this is done for you. You don't think about it. You don't direct this action. You lay back and enjoy the benefits.

In just the time taken to read this paragraph, your hair has grown, your finger and toe-nails are longer ... all this activity results from orderly communication from the brain (CNS) to cells making up the tissues and organs of your body.

How much work the brain does is made clear in that it needs three times more oxygen to develop energy than do other parts of the body. Oxygen is the prime ingredient in turning food into body energy.

Scientists are constantly discovering brain "centers," specialized cells which control specific functions, such as our "righting" reflex, which maintains the body's equilibrium—areas of hunger, thirst, temperature control and defense against invading noxious agents.

We are learning more about *endorphins*—brain substances which act like opiates. These little-known chemicals can kill pain in your body with the same effect as the drug morphine, a derivative of opium—*without the side effects.*

The brain is divided into two hemispheres, the right and the left.

The right side, it is believed, is responsible for dreams, abstract thoughts and irrationality.

The left side is concerned with the opposite: logic, verbal expression and rationality.

The spinal nerves, which connect with the brain and travel the length of the spinal column, are a division of the CNS.

These nerves exit the spinal cord through an opening between the vertebrae called *foramina*. When a vertebra is out of place, pressure is put upon the nerve, disrupting its smooth flow of energy at this irritated level of the spine.

Actually, a spinal nerve has two portions, the front, (*anterior*) and the back, (*posterior*) "root" (see Fig. 40).

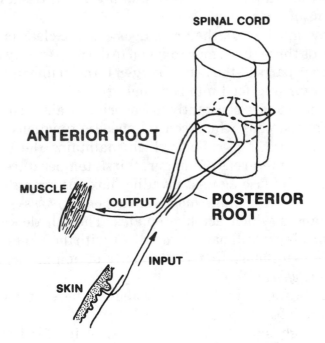

Fig. 40—Spinal nerves exit from an opening between the vertebra. There are two main branches of a nerve, the front (anterior) and back (posterior).

When a nerve receives stimulation from pressure—or from any disturbance in body function—the somatic fibers which control the musculo-skeletal parts of the body react with the painful symptoms associated with backache: sciatica, neuritis, bursitis, neuralgia and radiculitis.

The spinal root is that portion of the nerve alongside the vertebra. When a vertebra is out of its normal position—or alignment—with the vertebra above and below, you experience backache. This malalignment—a *subluxation*—narrows the opening and squeezes the tissues surrounding the nerve, causing immediate sharp and penetrating pain (Fig. 41).

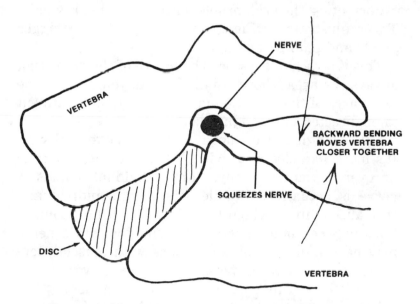

Fig. 41 demonstrates how bending backward too far can cause a pincer effect which creates pressure upon the nerve. Should the disc protrude backward, this pushes the posterior longitudinal ligament into the space occupied by the nerve. This reduction in diameter of the opening crowds the nerve, causing a painful reaction.

The spinal nerves actually are called the *peripheral nervous system*, because they convey impulses to organs and outlying parts of the body.

Sensations experienced by the body and organs are conveyed to the spinal cord and then to the brain via the spinal cord.

For a better understanding of the pathways of various nerves, consider two points:

One, pain in an elbow, for example, seldom originates at this site, unless you received a blow there. The pain starts from a condition in the neck and travels to the elbow by the *Ulner* spinal nerve, which transmits impulses to and from the elbow.

Correcting the neck problem relieves the elbow pain. This is illustrated in Figure 42, which shows the trigger points and pain patterns.

This is a valuable lesson. The source of the pain is not always the area where pain is felt. As you can see, the exact area of the irritation must be found for treatment to be directed to the right place.

Two, a single nerve is not a solid object, like steel wire. It's more like electrical wire. When the outer layer is uncovered, you find many, many individual strands. A nerve is actually a bundle of separate, individually specialized fibers which branch out with interconnections between other nerves. One fiber within a nerve may have hundreds of connections with muscles, tendons, ligaments, blood vessels and other nerves.

The following may clarify the nerve function:

Your big toe touches a hot object. A sensation of heat is sent to your brain. This impulse doesn't travel a straight line, like a string connecting your toe to your brain. Although it moves at lightning speed, it passes

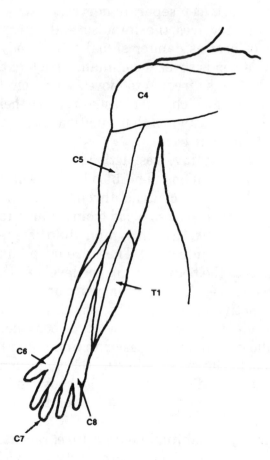

Fig. 42 shows the sensory areas of the arm supplied by spinal nerves which originate in the cervical and upper thoracic areas of the spine. The designations refer to the specific spinal nerves which supply energy to the arm area.

through several junctions *(synapses)*, where the urgency of the message is shared with other interconnecting nerve fibers. It ascends to the brain through a chain of the linkages between separate nerves.

The brain receives the impulse and interprets the sensation of heat as danger signal to the body. Simultaneously, it sends several commands back to the body.

First, the leg is directed to move away from the heat. The sequence in which other tissues receive their orders is unclear, but it is known that functions associated with defense of the body occur.

Leg movement involves action by muscles, bones, ligaments and tendons. The blood vessels in the area expand and leg veins contract through a milking action of muscles to drain excess blood from the area to prevent congestion. An increase in lymph fluid is supplied to combat possible infection. The adrenal glands squirt adrenalin into the body, raising the level of blood sugar to produce energy for emergency action.

All this activity is initiated by nerves, acting singly or interdependently over the network of body nerves.

The following makes it easier to understand how the pain of backache originating in the spine may be referred to a more distant part of the body, and how that part refers it back to the brain over the pathway of nerves (Fig. 43).

Pressure from habitual poor posture, repeated physical activity which violates proper body mechanics—such as improper lifting—and a jarring or compressive injury may move the spinal disc to an abnormal position. This disc pressure often refers pain into the rectal area. Reducing the irritation at the correct level in the spine can relieve the pain felt in the rectum, because the cause of the pressure has been resolved.

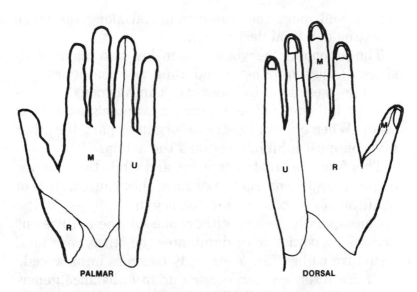

PALMAR DORSAL

Fig. 43 demonstrates the pattern of distribution of the Ulnar (U) and Radial (R) nerves which originate in the neck and supply nervous energy to the hand and arm.

NERVOUS ENERGY CAN KEEP YOU OFF-BALANCE

Another division of the nervous system is the autonomic nervous system, so-called because this functions involuntarily, without conscious thought on your part.

This system attends to the body's housekeeping chores. It provides a constant, regulated flow of energy from the brain to the heart, stomach, liver and other organs of digestion, the blood vessels, involuntary muscles, and body glands.

This system is responsible for making the heart pump, the stomach digest and the small intestines absorb nu-

97

trition and move the waste material along the large intestine to a final destination.

The autonomic nervous system has two major divisions, 1) the sympathetic and 2) parasympathetic.

While these two divisions work in harmony, the actions or influences of each division is antagonistic to the other. When one stimulates an organ or part, the other division must inhibit, or retard the action.

This function creates balance, and while these nerves do not literally control the organs, they cause a state of equilibrium to exist within the organ.

Consequently, when either one of these divisions becomes superactive or dominates the other, your total structure will suffer. Your body becomes imbalanced.

Organ disorders can occur due to imbalance generated by the overpowering influence of either division. You may check for symptoms by reviewing the chart at the end of this chapter which shows the effects of dominance by either the sympathetic or parasympathetic division.

The sympathetic system mobilizes the body in situations of fear and anger. Stress and tension, popularly known as the "Triple F" syndrome, trigger body defenses when a person is faced with a situation involving FRIGHT, FLIGHT or FIGHT.

What would you feel if someone held a gun to your head?

Fear, of course.

This sensation—of fear and anger—sets off many body adaptations: pupils dilate, blood vessels bring blood from internal organs to *peripheral* muscles, vessels supplying organs and digestive apparatus become constricted, heart beat increases, blood pressure goes up, the liver converts stored glycogen into blood sugar for immediate energy, the adrenal and thyroid glands secrete hormones to increase the metabolic rate, and your lungs pump faster and harder to produce a greater supply of the oxygen needed for tissue energy and nutrition.

Knowing how the sympathetic nervous system takes over when you are threatened gives you the power to divert emotional situations which throw your body into the Fight and Flight syndrome without compelling reason.

It's better not to give in to fear when backache occurs.

Infections also stimulate the sympathetic nervous system to arouse the body's defense mechanism. You're familiar with how rapidly your heart beats and how dry your mouth and skin become when temperature rises and how you lose appetite and become constipated with a decrease in action of intestinal muscles.

All these symptoms show the overpowering influence of the sympathetic nervous system.

The reverse action—good appetite, carefree digestion, easy elimination and increased sexual desire—are guided by the *parasympathetic* division of the *autonomic nervous system.*

Writers use effects of the nervous system to an advantage in describing "The sweet flush of success," "The ecstasy of passion" or "The agony of despair."

Here, again, is an example of how important balance is to the total well-being of the human body—and how you can use this knowledge to control the pain of backache.

When you're under seige with a backache, you can expect to be dominated by all the influences of the *sym pathetic* division of the *autonomic nervous system.*

During the investigation of your pain, remember the various ways a nerve root can produce pain: through stretching, compression, kinking, tearing, inflammation and irritation inflicted by repeated postural abuse, improper lifting, joint instability and violent body movements of contact sports, or ill-advised physical activity.

EFFECT OF DRUGS ON THE CNS

Many of my "first-time" patients express concern that they will receive no drugs—no pain killers or muscle relaxants—as part of their chiropractic program.

However, the initial apprehension usually disappears during our consultation.

"What type treatment have you received for your backache?" is my first question.

"Tranquilizers and muscle relaxers," is the usual response.

"Is that the only treatment you've received?"

"Yes. My doctor gave me this prescription and told me to check with him in two weeks."

"And you still have the back pain?"

"Yes."

Of course, it then becomes obvious to the patient that if drugs were doing the job intended, the backache would be gone—at least somewhere near resolution.

Many people are unaware of the distinction between the purely drug—medical—approach to backache with the drugless—chiropractic—method of correcting spinal problems and whip-lash injury.

100

Neither system, I believe, holds all the answers to all the ills people can devise. However, everyone should be aware of the existence of a form of treatment which is different from the orthodox approach in most medical estabishments.

It all melts down to this: which approach do you prefer for your backache or other musculo-neuro-skeletal problems—drugs which deaden pain and do nothing about the cause or causes? Or the non-drug methods which logically search out the anatomical physiological problems and deal with them?

Which is better for *you?*

Here's the standard medical treatment for backache and soft tissue damage: a prescription of the drug Valium (the most widely used) or Darvon, both of which block pain by depressing activity of the central nervous system.

According to many patients, the prescription is written without a thorough examination or inspection, other than x-rays, of the spine.

Synthetic narcotics such as Darvon, Percodan, Demerol and others are compounded from coal tar or petroleum products. Like opium and its derivatives, they are potentially addictive. Those who use them over a long period and try to quit go through the torment of withdrawal—an intense craving, intestinal distress, black depression, irritability and extreme nervousness.

These narcotics don't cure cells or tissues, muscles, bones, tendons, ligaments or blood vessels at the site of the injury. They merely deaden the symptoms.

Drugs can be dangerous—even deadly—in a life-threatening, physical emergency, especially when the attending doctor is not aware or alerted to the patient's

101

negative reaction to certain narcotics.

Another hazard of drugs, including Valium, is that they may mask the true physical condition and delay or make difficult an exact diagnosis. Then, too, interactions of certain drugs can cause serious complications.

Most chiropractors would adjust the spine of backache patients, if indicated. Purpose? To normalize the effect on injured tissues, muscles, ligaments and bones, removing the cause of pain and working to produce balance between the *parasympathetic* and *sympathetic* divisions of the *autonomic* central nervous system.

This is not to say every patient seeking care from a medical or chiropractic doctor would receive identical treatment or response. In California, for example, there are Holistic Health Clinics where care is provided by a team—medical and chiropractic doctors, nutritional and physical therapists.

Typically, how does the chiropractor deal with pain? By many processes other than drugs. Applied to the specific area of complaint, pain control is usually more effective over a longer period of time than the chemical, non-specific shotgun treatment which involves and affects organs and cells of the whole body.

Chiropractic is a wholly natural physical procedure which offers a package of plus factors: a thorough exam for strains, sprains, whiplash and other soft tissue injuries; drugless pain control applied to a specific area of complaint or other sources of the problem; guidance of the patient to self-help: posture correction, exercises and other ways of getting to the root of the problem; adjustments to correct disabling factors, and physical and emotional counsel to return the patient to wholeness and normal functioning.

While the drugs of a physician may deaden the pain of a broken arm bone, they will not mend the condition. A trained doctor must adjust the fractured bone to normal alignment, immobilize the arm and allow it to heal. Later several exercises and proper nutrition will rebuild muscle strength and control and restore normal movement.

Mineral levels in the blood stream and tissues are greatly affected by the effects of injury. These factors are discussed in detail in Chapter 7.

In finishing the comparison of medical doctors and chiropractors, it might be well to mention that countless lives have been seriously threatened—many ruined—through freely prescribed drugs for various physical conditions. Such cases range through the population from the well-known to the little-known.

For painful arthritis, Betty Ford, the former First Lady, was given a drug to which she became addicted, combining it with alcohol, another depressant.

Anita Bryant plunged herself into deep depression due to dependency upon tranquilizers and wine.

A letter-writer to Ann Lander's advice column allowed herself to become addicted to Valium because she was afraid to expose her feelings of "inadequacy." Her doctor helped develop this dependency by refilling prescriptions rather than assume the role of "physician," which, in its broader sense, means *teacher*.

Unfortunately, such examples of case mismanagement are not uncommon.

The magic of the word "balance" applies to all phases of our life.

Usually a common-sense approach to a problem brings everything necessary to provide the balance the body requires for optimum health.

That's why we started this chapter with the amazing nervous system, showing how pain is generated and why it sometimes shows up far away from the problem area, and then finished with a comparison of methods used by medical doctors and chiropractors.

There's more to come in the next chapter—mainly about how to bring an end to the pain and inconvenience of backache.

CHART OF THE PHYSIOLOGICAL ACTIONS OF THE AUTONOMIC NERVOUS SYSTEM

	SYMPATHETIC	*PARASYMPATHETIC*
Eye	Dilates pupil	Constricts pupil Facilitates accommodation
Lacrimal glands	Constricts blood vessels Inhibits secretion	Stimulates secretion
Mucous membranes of the head	Constricts blood vessels Inhibits secretion	Dilates blood vessels Stimulates secretion
Salivary glands	Increases the secretion of organic substances of the saliva and possibly constricts blood vessels	Increases the secretion of the watery elements of the saliva and possibly dilates the blood vessels
Thyroid gland	Vasomotor Increases secretion	Decreases secretion (?)
Heart	Accelerates heart rate, augments force of contraction and possibly dilates coronary arteries	Decreases rate, conductivity and force of contraction and constricts coronary arteries
Bronchi	Constricts blood vessels Inhibits secretion Relaxes bronchial muscles	Contracts bronchial muscles Increases secretion
Esophagus	Vasomotor	Contracts
Cardiac orifice	Vasomotor	Constricts and relaxes
Stomach	Constricts blood vessels Inhibits gastric motility Decreases secretion of HCl	Increases gastric motility Stimulates secretion of HCl
Pyloric orifice	Contracts	Relaxes

105

Organ		
Small intestine	Constricts blood vessels Inhibits peristalsis Decreases secretion	Stimulates peristalsis Increases secretion
Colon and rectum	Constricts blood vessels Inhibits peristalsis Decreases secretion Constricts anal sphincter	Stimulates peristalsis Increases secretion Relaxes anal sphincter
Pancreas	Inhibits secretion of pancreatic juice	Increases secretion of pancreatic juice
Spleen	Vasomotor Contracts smooth muscles of capsule and trabecula	Unknown
Liver	Vasomotor Converts glycogen into glucose, increases protein metabolism in liver, inhibits cholesterol secretion in the bile	Inhibits protein metabolism in the liver and increases cholesterol secretion in the bile
Gall bladder	Relaxes muscles of gall bladder and constricts sphincters of bile ducts	Contracts muscles of gall bladder wall
Adrenal gland	Vasomotor Increases secretion of adrenalin	
Kidney	Vasomotor	Unknown
Urinary bladder	Contracts muscles of trigone and sphincter Relaxes muscles of bladder wall	Relaxes muscles of trigone and sphincter Contracts muscles of bladder wall
Ovaries or testes	Vasomotor	
Fallopian tubes and uterus	Stimulates contraction of muscles of tubes and uterus	Probably activates cervix and inhibits contraction of body of uterus
Prostate gland	Vasomotor	Contracts muscles within gland
Penis and clitoris	Vasomotor	Causes erection

CHAPTER 5
Pain Control Combines Art
With Science

"Dr. Lindsey, why isn't there a better way to relieve pain than taking knock-out pills?" a female patient with a back problem asks.

"There is. The best way to avoid pain is to prevent it from occuring."

She didn't like this answer. Nobody does. Yet that's telling it like it is. A diabetic knows what sugar can do to him. An alcoholic realizes he can't take that first drink. The smoker who wants to quit is aware he can't light up.

All right, what are the rules for preventing pain? Here are some "how-to's":

1) Strengthen weak muscle groups which allow poor posture spinal curves and faulty body mechanics. (Figs. 3, 4 and 5).

2) Bend, sit and lift erectly as possible. That's how to avoid skeletal abuse, using body muscles in positions for which they were not designed (Fig. 44).

3) Sleep on a firm, supporting mattress.

4) Do the corrective exercises in this book—every other day, at least.

5) Avoid becoming overweight. A sag in the abdominal muscles permits organs to become displaced, displaces your center or gravity and sets you up for back strain.

6) Shun diet and drugs which make tissues oversensitive: sugar, salt (which causes water-retention); cigarettes, and the many drugs (including socially acceptable Valium and other tranquilizers) which bring on

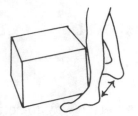

1. The Feet
The feet should be approximately 10-12 inches apart. Place one foot alongside the object to be lifted. The other foot should be placed to give the feeling of comfortable balance and stability. This will allow the body to be in a position for the upward thrust of the lift. If you have to turn with a load, change the position of your feet, do not twist the body.

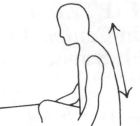

2. The Back
Keep the back straight. This helps keep the spine, muscles, and body organs in correct alignment. It also helps to alleviate some of the pressure which builds up in the abdominal region during lifting and can cause hernias and other types of strain.

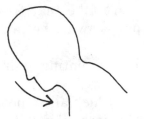

3. The Chin
The chin should be tucked in slightly so that the neck and spine continue in a straight line. This helps to reduce injuries to the neck region and aids in total spinal balance.

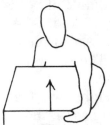

4. Arms and Elbows
Bring the object to be lifted as close to the body as possible. When arms are held away from the body, much strength is lost. The object becomes more difficult to lift because of a change in center of gravity. Spinal balance is greatly affected by proper position of the object. Many strains and sprains are caused by this imbalance.

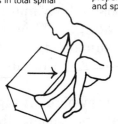

5. Body Position
The body position is essential in order to maintain proper weight distribution over the feet. This position also enables the body to better balance the weight and gives much easier ability to thrust during the lift. Keep loads as close to the body as possible.

(Courtesy "Introduction to Chiropractic", Dr. Sportelli, Palmerton, P.A.)

Fig. 44—How to lift properly.

muscle pain during withdrawal.

Prevention must be full-time, an all-out effort. It's a change in life-style, a switch from a backache sufferer to a non-sufferer.

Prevention is putting energy into your vitality account, off-setting the withdrawals of bad habits which drain your physical resources and cloud your mental perception.

In daily living, we can't always control the stress, tension and pressures of the world, but we *can* control our emotional reactions to them. Many repeated negative reactions can magnify our pain, which, in turn, makes our depression more heavy.

If our mental outlook says, "Everything is hopeless," the body agrees with a hanging head, dropping shoulders, a bowed back and a falling pelvis, which causes a sway in our low back.

No wonder we hurt!

To a stranger who views our external collapse, no surprise we're tagged as "losers"—we look the part.

The emotional imbalance resulting from lack of physical stamina leads to greater physical imbalance. Moving body parts which should be in harmony like instruments of a great symphony orchestra—bones, muscle, organs and blood vessels—are in discord, outside the laws of biomechanical logic. Discord means pain.

A small percentage of the thousands of bad back cases who have come to me in thirty years of chiropractic practice has experienced a peculiar twist of mind and emotions. *They actually did not want to get well!* They appeared to be enjoying their disability—dependency and the delicious attention paid to their physical needs—excuses for not conscientiously trying to clear up problems of body and mind.

Most back victims, however, earnestly want to be healed. Although some preventive measure can help them, they may need treatment from a doctor who understands the spine and the many obvious and hidden causes which can make a back ache.

Unfortunately most medical doctors are not schooled in handling such conditions. They only use the methods learned in their particular school of training—an arsenal of pills which deaden the pain and do nothing about the reasons for the pain. This is the best argument for bringing your back problem to someone who understands the spine and the structures which create your pain.

Fortunately for the public there is movement in the direction of educational seminars which invite, and are attended by, practitioners of all disciplines, MD, DC, DO and DDS. Subjects range from acupuncture to meditation, nutrition to pain control. The emphasis is toward providing the patient all modes of care which will restore health, not provide physical and emotional crutches. The underlining is the patient must be responsible for his health and must understand the mechanism responsible for creating a condition of ill-health, pain and the emotionally crippling effects of dependency.

I have seen many patients who have come to me in desperation after prolonged medical treatment with drugs for their back problem. Not only did they still have their bad back but also a drug habit. They had progressed up the potency scale from mild tranquilizers to stronger formulae and more frequent dosages. Natural or synthetic drugs which depress the cental nervous system are taken by mouth, injected into the bloodstream via a muscle or beneath the skin at the point of pain. After repeated use, they depress the patient and give him or her a feeling of hopelessness.

One successful chiropractor refuses to treat patients who have undergone treatment with cortisone or other steroids. He believes use of these drugs so depresses the normal metabolic activity that restoring the patient's prior vitality is not possible.

All right. If most medical doctors cannot or do not get to the root of the problem, where can I turn? To the man or woman who is skilled in relieving back pain—the local chiropractor. For more than eighty years, licensed and qualified chiropractors have made spinal adjustments and given related treatments for such conditions. They succeed by reducing pressure on spinal nerves—the most common cause for pain in muscles, ligaments and the skeleton.

There is no known substitute for adjusting a misaligned vertebra, rib or joint of the skeleton. The contributing editors of this book—many of them eminent in their profession—have recommended corrective exercises which, if practiced, will stabilize mechanical problems. These are presented later in this chapter and in chapter 8.

Another approach to relieving pain is restoring normal blood circulation in the area of pain. Blood and fluids accumulate in the tissues. This stagnant, pooling prevents or limits the flow of fresh, healing blood to the area. Heat applications, rhythmic galvanic current, ultrasound and massaging can disperse pooling. Massaging mimics the milking action of muscles required to move blood in the veins from the injured zone. It literally draws in fresh blood.

The secret of recovery from backache lies in getting

111

to the specific cause of the pain. And while swelling may be producing the pain, you must determine the factors which precipitate this swelling. There are many causes for irritation—toxic secretions from tissues called *catobolites*, infective agents, spurs of mineral deposits which jab into surrounding tissues, stretching the root of a spinal nerve, or a squeezed disc which is pushing into the back and putting a kink in the (posterior) spinal ligament. (Fig. 45"D").

Pain relieving medications accomplish no basic structural change, they rely upon correction through self-limiting means. Since there is no alteration in the defective structure, the condition progresses in its destructive activity.

There's no panacea, no magic wand to wipe out the ache of irritated muscles, ligaments and nerves of the broad back. Not even chiropractic adjustments work in every case.

Harry G., a truck driver for a large grocery chain, is an example of what can happen to the body by disregarding the evidence of existing structural damage.

From x-rays, Harry was aware of a congenital defect—a *spondylolisthesis* (a sliding forward of the fifth lumbar vertebra away from the adjacent sacrum and fourth lumbar vertebra). (Fig. 45"C").

Harry was warned against lifting—any lifting—as this could cause additional slippage of the vertebra and increase pressure upon the disc to the point of rupture.

"I can't change jobs, Doc. I owe too much money to take a lower paycheck."

So, Harry went with the money but an accident at work pushed his back to the near breaking point. After two surgeries, Harry was still in a wheel chair, totally destitute, both financially and physically. A third sur-

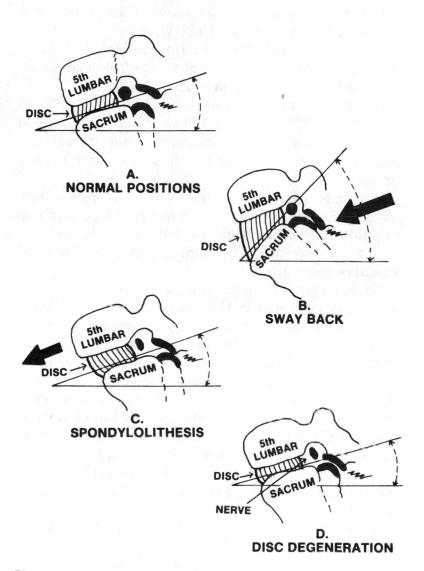

**A.
NORMAL POSITIONS**

**B.
SWAY BACK**

**C.
SPONDYLOLITHESIS**

**D.
DISC DEGENERATION**

Fig. 45—The normal alignment of A) is contrasted by unbalanced posture. The "pelvic tilt" exercise can relieve strain on this fifth lumbar and sacrum joint.

113

gery to fuse the bones in his spine was Harry's only hope to return to even minimal employment.

There is no benefit realized from neglect. Sometimes however, a patient may just run out of patience in attempting to find a solution to their problem.

If your doctor's treatment has been unsuccessful and he tells you, "The pain is all in your head," it's time to head for another doctor. A more sympathetic and eager practitioner may discover the elusive solution to your problem.

But understand one thing: there's seldom a purely black and white solution or an A to Z scientific roadmap to guide your doctor right to the source of your complaint. It's *your* pain. Give him or her all the help and guidance you can.

Never forget that medicine is called "the healing arts" for a very good reason. Getting people well challenges every known human resource on occasion—gut reaction, horse-sense, science and mother nature. The bottom line is, healing is a balance between art and science.

The more you understand about the behavior of your body tissues, the better chance you have to help in reducing pain. An example of your body's interactions is shown in Chapter 2, a sketch of the cycle of pain. I'm not suggesting that everyone can succeed with even the best outlined aching back "do-it-yourself" project. I believe it's worth a try, but if you don't succeed turn to a practitioner.

It's a tribute to the warmth and sympathy of people that they want to help—kindly relatives, neighbors, or some person who "had the very same thing." While many individuals have experienced pain from backache, rarely does anyone have the "very same thing" you have.

114

There are too many variables possible for this to happen. "Everybody is a little different" is more than a cliche. It is solid truth. You react differently to physical stress than I do. Your tolerance to pain is more or less than mine. Your response to chemicals, physical and emotional stimulus is as exclusive to you as your fingerprints (see Chapter 1). So the best thing to do is accept advice from these well-intentioned persons with appreciation and resolve to keep from making your aching back a "Gong Show" rerun or an amateur production. Free advice is worth every penny you pay for it. Turn to a professional who is trained in this field.

THREE POSTURAL POSITIONS

Meanwhile, learn everything you can about your condition through the three postural position tests—standing, sitting and moving (Fig. 46). When you don't conform to standards shown, you can bet your posture is causing stress somewhere in your musculo-skeletal system. You can also bet that you've got a backache as a result.

Remember that when you stand correctly, your body is supported in the front by the *anterior* (front) ligament and in the back by the *posterior* (back) ligament. These strong fibrous bands parallel the spinal column (Fig. 47). If your body relied solely on muscles to hold it in

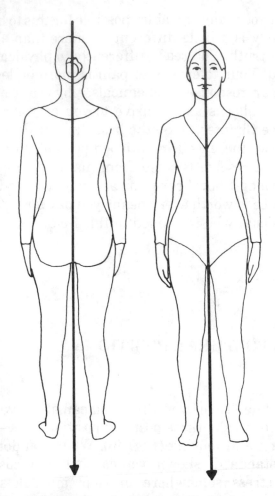

Fig. 46—An example of perfect posture. To analyze your posture, visualize a vertical line that runs through the ear . . . through the shoulder . . . midway through the chest . . . through the hip . . . through the knee . . . and through the ankle. This is the role-model children should adopt to develop their posture. When begun early in life, good posture becomes a fixed habit. Every home and classroom should display a Perfect Posture Chart to train children in this important aspect of body and health development. Every adult should use the Perfect Posture Chart daily to gain awareness of healthful benefits of improved posture.

116

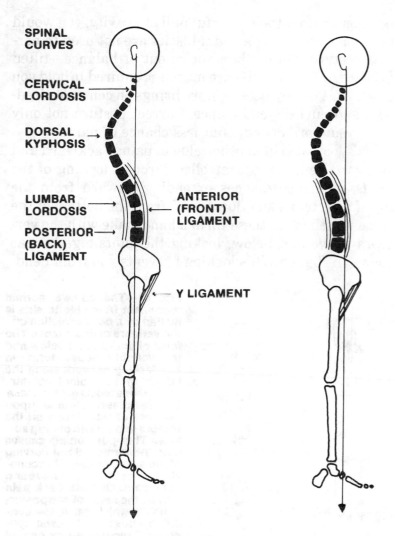

SPINAL
CURVES

CERVICAL
LORDOSIS

DORSAL
KYPHOSIS

LUMBAR
LORDOSIS

ANTERIOR
(FRONT)
LIGAMENT

POSTERIOR
(BACK)
LIGAMENT

Y LIGAMENT

Fig. 47—The relaxed, upright body stance should be supported by ligamentous support, not by contracting muscles. If you experience unusual fatigue, perhaps you're overworking muscles. The plumb line shows the correct positioning of the body to maintain harmony with the forces of gravity with upright posture. It is strain on the posterior (back) ligaments which travel along the spine which cause back pain. The front (anterior) ligaments are not imbued with the identical pain-producing fibers as the posterior ligaments.

117

position against the powerful pull of gravity, you would be exhausted by day's end. Muscles are not used in normal posture. Only when you're out of balance—tilted forward or backward—are muscles required to hold you erect. This is why poor posture brings on constant tiredness and curtails endurance. Correct posture not only gives you more energy, but less chance of pain.

Let's look at still another clue to pain. Backward and sideward bending is controlled through locking of the *facets*, ingenious devices extending upward from the top of a vertebra and downward from the bottom of the same vertebra . . . these form a handshake with the vertebra above and below, locking the joints together, as shown in Fig. 48. This locking prevents you from bend-

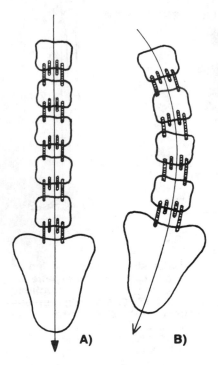

A)   B)

Fig. 48—The spine's normal movement from side to side is limited by a bony projection on the vertebra called a facet. The facet of the vertebra below and the vertebra above form an interlocking network along the length of the spinal column. When these facets get too close together pressure is made upon the sacs of fluid found on the facets's joining and gliding surface. This positioning causes pain. Abnormal lateral curving of the spine, as found in scoliosis, causes facetal pressure and back pain. Chronic back pain may be the result of bad postural habits which cause the condition known as "facetal syndrome," recognized by painful bending and constant aching of the lower back. The action of bending, twisting, stooping and turning requires a certain "rhythmic" movement of the involved structures. When motion is limited due to mal-

aligned facets (and vertebrae) the normal rhythm of movement is distorted, causing additional strain to muscles and ligaments. An athlete may find his total potential far below normal due to even a slight disturbance in this normal pelvic rhythmic execution.

ing backward or sideward too far. If you tend to lean a little backward, you're putting extra—unnatural—weight on the *facets* and drawing them together. Over a long period of time you will bring on a cluster of pain, a condition known as *facet syndrome*.

Whenever your sitting, standing or moving is imbalanced, you cause stress, confirmed by pain. Effects of imbalanced posture are cumulative. The longer you put up with bad structural alignment, the more likely you are to invite pain. A simple explanation of this is supplied through:

LINDSEY'S LAW OF DEFICIT BALANCE

Imagine you have $100.00 in the bank. If you make regular withdrawals without depositing more money, sooner or later, you will end up with a zero balance. That's the way it is with your body. You arrive in the world with a given potential of physical stamina, energy, power—your *total energy quotient*.

Everyday you make withdrawals from your energy bank account. Every day you should be making deposits into it—good posture, exercise, nutritious foods, adequate rest and sleep, a relaxing hobby, an emotional life which gratifies, rather than frustrates, a positive mental outlook, a friendly and loving attitude. You can bankrupt your total energy quotient by doing just the opposite—pursuing a body-bruising or maiming occupation like Evel Knievel, you can live entirely on fast-foods and get habituated to alcohol or narcotics.

If both your parents died at an early age, this may signal you that your individual power supply is less than those individuals with obvious physical endurance, such as men who run several miles daily at the age of 60, 70 even 85. Ivor Welch completed the Colorado Peaks Marathon at age 85. Floridian Tom Gaskins jogged 10 miles on his 71st birthday.

As Ann Landers writes, "The train goes in both directions."

Each day of your life, you should make deposits to offset withdrawals—particularly during holiday seasons when overindulgence is difficult to avoid.

If you deplete your account prematurely, expect a notice from your banker—a backache, which reminds you to straighten up with a deposit, or suffer the pain of bankruptcy.

Although impending bankruptcy doesn't usually show up in your youth, it can happen even in the early years. As an example, consider the sway back, the most common mechanical cause for back pain. As a developing, young adult, you may withstand spinal imbalance, because you have youth and strength going for you—a large, untapped balance in your energy account.

Should you do heavy physical work with an imbalanced spine, you will drain your remaining balance quicker than normal (Fig. 49). And this means living a longer period of time with chronic back pain.

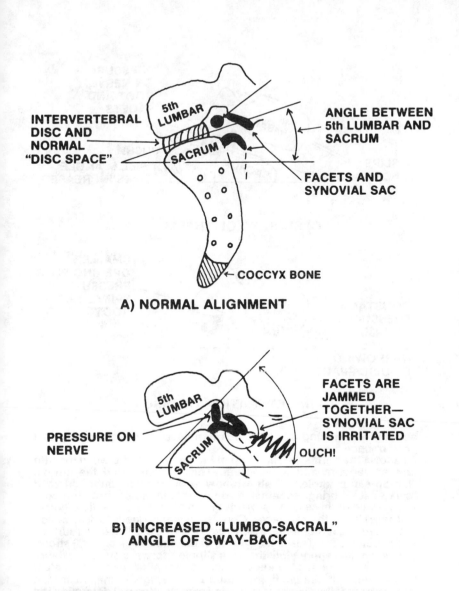

INTERVERTEBRAL DISC AND NORMAL "DISC SPACE"

5th LUMBAR

ANGLE BETWEEN 5th LUMBAR AND SACRUM

SACRUM

FACETS AND SYNOVIAL SAC

← COCCYX BONE

A) NORMAL ALIGNMENT

5th LUMBAR

FACETS ARE JAMMED TOGETHER— SYNOVIAL SAC IS IRRITATED

PRESSURE ON NERVE

SACRUM

OUCH!

B) INCREASED "LUMBO-SACRAL" ANGLE OF SWAY-BACK

Fig. 49—Parents who witness development in their children of "sway" back may dismiss the importance of this on-going structural abnormalcy because "it runs in the family." There is no valid reason to allow this physical imperfection to continue "running." You can put the brakes on the progress of this developing low back curve with proper remedial measures suggested in Chapter 3 and Chapter 8. Or, have the child x-rayed and follow the advice of a spinal specialist, who can

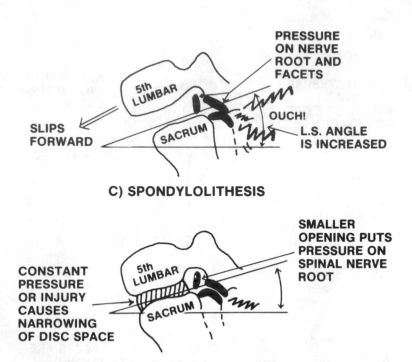

C) SPONDYLOLITHESIS

PRESSURE ON NERVE ROOT AND FACETS

SLIPS FORWARD

OUCH!

L.S. ANGLE IS INCREASED

5th LUMBAR

SACRUM

SMALLER OPENING PUTS PRESSURE ON SPINAL NERVE ROOT

CONSTANT PRESSURE OR INJURY CAUSES NARROWING OF DISC SPACE

5th LUMBAR

SACRUM

D) DEGENERATION OF DISC

assist in eliminating this insidious handicap which lowers physical performance.

A) shows the normal relationship of the facet space between the fifth lumbar vertebra and the sacrum. This is considered the normal "lumbo-sacral angle." B) shows how an increased lumbar curve, a "sway back," brings together these opposing facets, irritating both the surface of these bony projections and the tiny sac of fluid (synovial sacs) lining their surfaces. Constant irritation leads to destruction of the sac and its contents. Also it roughens the cartilagenous surface of the bony facet. This is the source of constant back pain. C) shows a defect called spondylolisthesis, a slipping forward on one vertebra on another. This is also known as a "congenital" or "birth" defect which occurs in the faulty formation of the spine. In many cases, it passes from father to son. Only x-ray examination will determine the presence of this potentially troublesome anomaly. A person with this condition should not engage in heavy lifting, diving, or occupations or pursuits which involve repeated jarring or excessive use of back muscles. The pinching effect on a spinal nerve, which produces exquisite pain, is shown in D). This is caused by narrowing or degeneration of a disc occuring between vertebra.

Some macho men ignore their pain. It's unmanly to feel pain, they foolishly think. Maybe they deny its existence through aspirins. If they ignore or deaden pain, there's nothing to worry about. This assumption is usually false—painfully false.

Constant irritation—treated or untreated—stimulates the tissue buildup of mineral deposits. That's the body's natural chemical defense mechanism. Should these minerals form a bridge between two poorly positioned vertebrae, it is almost impossible to realign them to a non-irritating state without surgery. This problem condition will cause pain at that site or possibly transmit it to another part of the body—persistently.

Overdrawing the energy bank account with a habitual postural defect leads to sway back *(lumbar lordosis)*. The lower area of the spine shows more than the normal forward curve. This condition occurs when the pelvis inclines in a rotating movement forward and downward on one side and upward and backward on the other side (an *oblique movement*). As the curve increases with time, a curve higher in the spine must also occur to maintain balance. This double curving action shifts the center of gravity away from its desirable center—near the level of the second lumbar vertebra.

As the lumbar curve increases, the locking devices of the lumbar spine come closer together than they should, putting pressure on the *facets*—mentioned earlier—and on the small sacs of lubricating fluid lining their surfaces (Fig. 49).

Even that's not the end of the story. This exaggerated low back curve causes a narrowing of the opening through which spinal nerves exit (Fig. 49). Pressure on the nerve and surrounding tissues causes excrutiating pain and marked loss of ability to bend the spine forward, or sideward on the side of the curve.

Just how would a person get rid of painful backache generated by a forward sloping pelvis? By an easy, yet effective exercise done in bed before arising in the morning or going to sleep at night.

Lie on your back and pull upward from the pelvis (Fig. 24). As you lower abdominal muscles gain strength, try flexing your knees and coming off the flat surface of the bed—or floor—about six to twelve inches.

Remember to keep your buttocks tucked under. A buttock that hangs will allow the low back to bend. The object is to keep the low back flat, taking out the sway.

Your *lumbar lordosis* is partly due to weakness in the lower abdominal muscles and is not corrected by having a strong back.

In fact, a strong person develops the habit of lifting everything in sight without regard for proper mechanics . . . and his suffering is postponed. But, this disregard for bioengineering principles will pay-off with backache, sooner or later.

Remember, keep the pelvis tilted upward, the low back flat.

Once you master this procedure lying flat on your back, try holding your pelvis up while standing, walking and sitting. Yes, it feels strange at first. Obviously, if the low back condition has been with you for many years, a sudden change from what has become "normal" will give you a sensation of "different." This is because the body accommodates even to bad habits.

In time, your new, aligned and pain-free posture will become second nature and comfortable. Then returning to your former imbalanced self will really jolt you

(Fig. 50).

Pain and tension in the neck, upper back, shoulders and arms is due to the second most common postural fault—a forward head carriage. This can be seen by an observer from your side view. Your head and ear is forward of your shoulder (Fig. 51).

Your ear should be in line with your shoulder. Have someone else check your head carriage, because it's difficult to recognize imperfection in yourself. This cardinal sin of posture makes the shoulders sag downward and forward, causing the rib cage to be depressed. The ribs now slant more vertically, when they should flare out horizontally.

A compressed rib cage pushes the heart out of normal position into a downward slant, causing a tug on the vessels of the aorta, the great vessel above the heart, and its attachments. The result could be shortness of breath, chest and upper back pain, tension headache, decreased vitality and stamina.

You can turn this bad habit around easily in minutes a day. Stand flat against a wall, making certain your heels are snug to the wall, and pull backward into the wall. Touch your shoulders and back of your head to the wall, making sure that your chin is tucked in both downward and backward.

Probably the most glaring error in this exercise is raising your head and eyes, believing that your chin is going backward. To eliminate this possibility, look at an object in front of you on the same level as your eyes. If you find yourself looking up, you're not doing the exercise properly.

A suggestion for short people who tend to bend their head backward while talking to a taller person: Take a

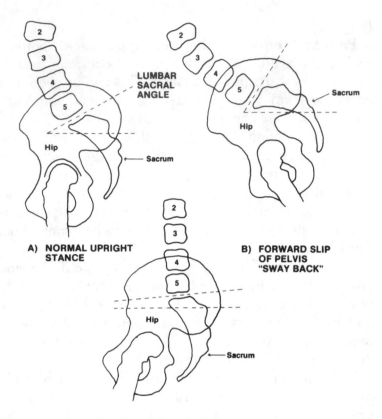

LUMBAR SACRAL ANGLE

2
3
4
5

Hip

Sacrum

A) NORMAL UPRIGHT
   STANCE

2
5
4
5

Sacrum

Hip

B) FORWARD SLIP
   OF PELVIS
   "SWAY BACK"

2
3
4
5

Hip

Sacrum

C) LOSS OF NORMAL CURVE
   BACKWARD TILT
   AND ABNORMAL
   MUSCLE TENSION
   RESULTING FROM INJURY

Fig. 50—Watch and feel your back symptoms disappear when you restore normal alignment in the angle between the fifth lumbar vertebra and the sacrum. If you allow "tilting" of the pelvis, you distort the foundation for your total postural support and gravitational alignment. A) Normal position of the spine and pelvis. B) Downward "tilt" of the pelvis and increased lower back curve. C) Decreased lumbar angle, "Flattening," causes abnormal straightening of the lumbar lordosis. Auto accidents, strains and other injuries can cause loss, or a reversing, of the normal back curvature.

126

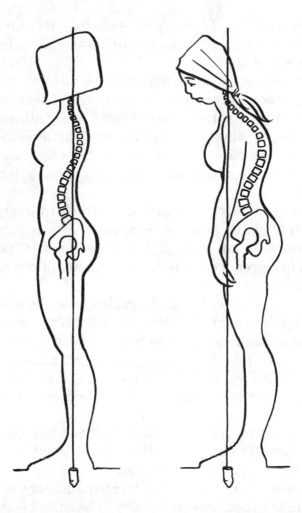

Fig. 51—How faulty posture causes pain in the neck. Carrying the head downward of the proper center of gravity causes the shoulders to fall forward and downward and the mid-back to bend backward into a kyphosis. This attitude is the typical slouched position. It causes downward pressure on the diaphragm and reduced capacity in the lungs. This common postural fault can be responsible for shoulder and neck pain. Continual forward head carriage can result in degeneration of the cervical disc and low back pain due to forward dropping of the pelvis.

127

step backward and direct your eyeballs—not your chin—upward. Keep your head and chin level without bending your neck (Fig. 52).

Just like the rest of us, athletes develop unwanted pain through poor posture. For the same reason, they perform under their potential. I have known many athletes who have upped their performances dramatically with improved posture. The difference between sub-power and super-power, between winning and losing, is correct stance.

Dr. Leroy Perry, a Pasadena, CA, chiropractor, has treated Olympic athletes from many countries and he has proven that even slight corrections in postural faults has produced outstanding results in competitive efforts.

A story in Good Earth Magazine tells about an incident which occurred during the 1979 Norman Manley Games in Jamaica. Alberto Juantoreno, a two-time gold medalist in the Montreal Olympics, was not supposed to run that day. He had dropped out of the 400 meter race, his best event, because of "mysterious" pains in his legs and lower back.

The Cuban team doctors were baffled by his condition, so *El Caballo* sought out Perry, who is called "Magic Fingers" by the hundreds of athletes he attends. After a quick examination, Perry treated Juantoreno with a technique called kinetic therapy to balance his muscles and reduce the stress in his hamstrings.

El Caballo got up from the training table and breezed to a first place finish in the 400. After breaking the tape he rushed across the infield and lifted the doctor into the air in celebration.

Perry demonstrates every day that balance can be the

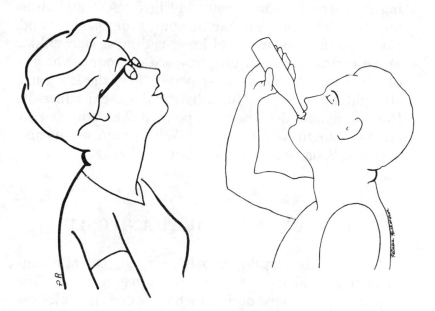

Fig. 52—Avoid bending the head backward. This saves wear on the cervical discs.

difference between first and second place, between competing or sitting on the sidelines.

Runners benefit immeasurably from a balanced posture, simply by being aware of feeling erect, rather than falling forward or backward from natural gravitational forces.

If you run in competition or just for fun, balance can add miles to your endurance. To make sure you're in balance have a partner observe you as you run past him or her. Do this several times. Still or motion pictures can also show exactly how erect you are.

If you would rather walk than run, be just as conscious about your upright stance. Imagine that you're imitating the correct posture shown in Fig. 53. A straight line must extend from your ear through your shoulder and chest, through the hip, and knee, ending at your ankle. Make certain that you pull upward on your lower abdominal muscles to lift your pelvis. Feel the low back straighten and flatten. Initially you'll sense tiredness in the tummy, but don't be disappointed. This only demonstrates your present weakness. With practice, this disappears. Soon you'll be outdistancing backache.

CHOOSING BETWEEN HEAT AND COLD

Temporarily, jogging or brisk walking can often aggravate a bad back. Then you want instant relief. This happened to a friend of mine who skidded on wet leaves

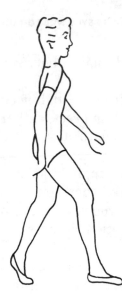

Fig. 53—Correct posture is necessary for walking and running as well as standing. Runners report an increase in speed and endurance following adaptation of better postural attitudes.
(Courtesy of Cervical Syndrome, Ruth Jackson, M.D., Charles C Thomas, Springfield, Ill).

while jogging in the dark.

"Dr. Dave, what should I use?" he asked. "A hot or cold compress?"

Like my friend, many people are confused on this subject. For acute trauma or injury, a *cold* application should be used quickly on the affected area.

If you own an ice-bag, utilize it. If you don't, wrap ice-cubes in a dish towel and apply them to the injured zone. Surround this with a large, dry bath towel to keep water from dripping over your body and on the floor. Commercial cold packs, reusable by refreezing, are inexpensive and easy to apply. Professional teams minimize the pain and damage of strains and sprains with them. Pro and amateur athletes wrap an arm, leg or elbow with them after sustained and vigorous workouts. This treatment can help runners avoid shin-splint pain.

Your objective is to reduce swelling.

Cold reduces swelling. *Swelling causes pain.* Remember also to elevate the injured part, if possible, to encourage the drainage of pooled blood from damaged tissues. Cold therapy decreases metabolism and increases blood circulation. One of the functions of blood is maintaining constant body temperature.

Treat the injured area—or painful area of backache—for 20 to 30 minutes, three to five times daily.

Heat is soothing relief for sore muscles and backache. However, heat also draws blood into the area, but does not constrict tiny capillaries in the area, as does cold. To prevent or reduce the accumulation of fluids in tissues—and alleviate pain—massage helps immeasurably. Light goading with the thumbs over the affected part is beneficial. Just stroke lightly—always in the

131

direction of the heart to return blood to this organ—and watch the swelling disappear.

Added to hot water bottles, diathermy and infrared heat lamps are effective heat producers. The hydrocullator treatment with hot packs and other heat producing equipment applied to injured and painful zones are helpful for temporary relief.

HOW TO PREVENT BACK STRAIN

How do back problems begin? In any number of ways.

Most athletic injuries occur early in the season, when bodies are not fully prepared for strenuous physical exertion commonplace with getting into shape.

Eagerness to beat the competition and anticipation of the upcoming season are factors which must be subdued early in training to allow gradual development of muscles and sufficient limberness to take the body joints to their maximum limit of movement.

Industrial injuries to the back frequently happen when the worker lifts improperly or when he is in an awkward position, standing on an uneven surface—a slope—or trying to catch a heavy weight while off balance.

Every chiropractor's file is filled with the worker's excuse for performing physical acts which were done against better judgment. Earl's case—similar to histories in every chiropractor's experience—was typical of the construction worker whose physical strength is actually his worst enemy. He always is in too much of a hurry to "get the job done." He can't wait for help from other crew members.

This bear of a man was a frequent visitor to the office. "Well, Earl, what happened this time?" He was doubled over with painful muscle spasm; both hands were gripping his thighs to make walking possible.

"I was lifting this wall when I felt a sharp pain in my back."

Carpenters build the wall frame flat on the ground and when it is completed several workers bend over and lift the wall to a vertical position. Earl became impatient and lifted a whole wall by himself and held it in position while a helper tacked it into place. It was too much for one man—a foolish thing to do.

"Earl, when will you stop giving your back to the company store?" I asked. "Just because you're strong as three oxen, is no reason to treat your back so disrespectfully."

"Well, Doc, I know you can get me over this. I guess I'm just going to slow down in the future . . . I can't afford many more of these situations, I lose too much work staying home with a bad back."

Chiropractors, orthopedic doctors, and work compensation insurance companies realize the advantages of prevention over treatment. Each injury—such as back strain—which tears some portion of the tendon or muccles away from its bony anchorage is repaired naturally with scar tissue. Just like a scar on the skin after a cut, this thick layer of connective tissue replaces the previously elastic tissue of the joint. Now—following injury—there remains this permanent residual of injury—setting up either an unstable joint likely to flop around and become easily displaced, or a joint so super-firm it cannot bend to its prior limits. Therefore, when activity demands movement at this joint, your mind responds but the joint can't supply the range you expect, consequently, another strain occurs due to taking the joint beyond its functional limit.

Several occurances of this kind may lead to *permanent disability* and retirement from construction and other types of industrial work requiring manual lifting or repeated standing in one position to perform tasks such as nailing, welding, soldering, painting and other similar occupations.

These are the ABC's of effective and safe lifting:

1) Bend and lift with both the back and legs straight **(Pg. 242). Too many workers strain back muscles by** bending forward from the hips when lifting or raising a heavy load with arms extended, away from the body. The latter method increases the load factor many times. A 25-pound box may be equivalent of 100 pounds in actual load stress.

To lift, bend both knees and lower your body with a straight back—a way of putting the power of the legs and back muscles into harmonious unison and avoiding back strain. Keep both arms close to your body with back erect.

During repeated lifting, try alternating your arms from right to left to distribute your muscle work.

Carpenters, when lifting walls, often bend forward almost to their toes, before starting to lift—as mentioned earlier, a procedure which often ends with painful strain and, over the years, contributes to chronic backache—and loss of income.

Even vacuuming the floors of a home in a bending-forward position can provoke many a backache and turn a relatively straight-forward bit of house-cleaning into a dreaded chore.

Many women are not aware of the principle of the vacuum cleaner, which moves dirt into the bag through air movement, not from a scrubbing action on the carpet. In many instances, you will find the dirt easier to pick up by gently lifting the carpet tool upward—rather than pushing downward on the floor tool. Stand up straight and let the vacuum do the job it was designed for.

Janice, an attractive secretary in her mid-twenties, came to see me for tension in her neck and upper back.

"I've got more tension in my back than warts on a toad," she said.

"You share this problem with thousands of other secretaries," I replied. "What the office world needs is a ten-minute relaxation break, rather than the so-called "rest period" or "coffee break."

"My boss would never go for that. All they want at my job is work, work and more work."

While this is true in Janice's case, many employers and office supervisors profit with increased production by following the successful pattern established in Japan which affords employee's time for mid-morning and afternoon "exercise." This productive period clears mind and body, actually increasing a person's ability to perform routine tasks, the repetition of which causes a form of mental and physical hypnosis and lack of concentration on the job being performed. When a person is mentally escaping from his present environment, the job can suffer as a consequence.

Short periods of physical exercise stimulates the entire body. Oxygen consumption is increased, stagnant fluids get shunted around and out, muscles get warm and relaxed and the brain comes back into focus. With increased body strength, it's easier to support the body in an erect and attentive attitude.

Secretaries, typists, draftspersons, desk workers—writers, accountants, attorneys and administrators—fall into the habit of craning their neck and cervical spine forward for several hours daily. Result? Tension headache, shoulder and neck pain and tightness—often the forerunners which, over the years, create back pain via degeneration—wearing out before its time—of the discs between the neck vertebra. You can do something to prevent immediate discomfort and future serious problems:

Take an occasional break. Let yourself go. Relax. Allow your head to rotate in a full circle—clockwise to counter-clockwise—several times . . . let the neck muscles go limp as cooked spaghetti.

Stand up and straighten up. Pull both shoulders back as far as you can. Elevate your chest (diaphragm) and take one or two deep breaths.

Rather than detract from production, this exercise break will add to it. Most errors are committed late in the afternoon, due to mental and physical fatigue and boredom. The more frequently you can break the fatigue cycle, the greater will be your output.

Many attorneys I know are not available in their office from noon to three o'clock. This used to annoy me until I discovered what was happening. They were all playing racquetball at the local physical fitness center!

"How can you afford to take this time from your office?" I asked my attorney.

"You make it sound like a penalty," he said. "In truth, it's not . . . it's benefit. I find I can accomplish twice the work I was doing before in about one-third the time.

Physically I feel so much better, my workload has increased but I have more stamina than ever before. Why don't you join us sometime? You'll feel the same way we do about our attitude toward work—it's a piece of cake."

With the daily practice of good posture, your back and abdominal muscles become stronger, allowing you to stand, sit and walk without straining muscles which have no business keeping you erect. For good behavior, your body will reward you less muscle cramping, annoying tension and general discomfort. The secret is awareness, a guaranteed good-habit-builder.

Using lightweight dumbbells (five pounds) to develop arm, shoulder and back muscles will increase above-the-waist strength and decrease chances of strain.

Using a slant-board (Fig. 54) five to ten minutes daily, especially at night before bedtime, will improve brain and upper body circulation and promote relaxation.

For general toning of the lower half of the body, walking briskly will improve foot, leg and thigh muscles and keep your ligaments elastic—important in preventing strain.

Exercises and body movements which stretch the back, legs and upper body—see Chapter 8—make for better muscle tone—the first and best defense against strain and pain.

It is important to remember this book is *not* a guide to Physical Fitness—it is a book dealing with specific conditions which cause backache and joint pain. (My book on the subject of fitness and general good health, *Dr. Lindsey's Ten Minute System for Perfect Health* is to be published later). Consequently, it is wise to know certain exercises—which may be good fitness builders—are bad medicine for certain back conditions. It's like "one man's

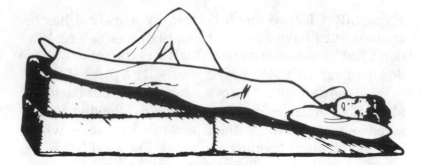

Fig. 54—A slant-board improves circulation by increasing circulation to head, shoulders and upper back areas. Additionally, it allows the spine to stretch without working at it, in fact, it can add inches to your total heighth. Another advantage is slanting downward allows organs to return to their natural positions. With a slant-board you experience sag-free posture.

meat is another man's poison" type of reasoning. You must only perform exercises and movements which help your *specific condition* without aggravating it. The few suggestions presented in this chapter were, or should be applicable for all persons, even those with specific back problems. But, do not attempt to engage in any program without advance knowledge the exercises being done will benefit your exact condition.

LITTLE THINGS CAN HURT

Pain is not always the result of big events in our lives ... little things can hurt, too. Insignificant factors of daily living—called stressors in the text book—can add up to big pain in the back, and elsewhere.

Just reaching over for an object on the floor can wallop

you good.

A weak body translates into negative emotions—lack of energy, lack of confidence, a feeling of inferiority and desire to stop the world and get off. Weak muscles tell your emotions to beg off from invitations to take a walk, go to a picnic, play 18-holes of golf, or join a bowling team.

The more flabby the muscular structure we live in, the more we withdraw from social life. And, living in isolation compounds the effects of emotional stress, which often ends up in backache or pain traveling through the body joints.

Physical fitness translates into positive emotions. What a small price to pay for emotional independence and constitutional invulnerability! You build a personal temple from indestructable materials designed for an eternity of blessed happiness!

Want to begin? And strengthen your body the easy way—without a rigid program of regulated exercises? Try the following:

1) If you sit while you work, plan a spare-time activity that calls for vigorous movement, such as square dancing. Some people follow a hobby that's as physically inactive as their gainful employment.

2) Stop being one sided. If your job calls for muscular movement on just the right side of your body, learn to switch to the opposite side, promote balance of body use, and prevent a lateral spinal curve from forming.

3) Put your body through a delightful variety of movement: skipping rope, jogging-in-place, handball, softball, tennis, swimming (but not the breast stroke with a sway back). Join a health club where you can watch your improvement in relation to others.

139

4) Perhaps you drive a lot. If so, walk more to offset the sameness in back position. Vary even your driving posture with a wedge-shaped cushion for your back.

5) If your work chair pushes into your lower back—adjust it to distribute pressure to the *entire* lower back—the upper as well as the lower lumbar vertebrae. The so-called secretarial chairs with "lumbar support" may cause a forward bending in the low back, a certain cause for back strain.

6) Replace worn shoes often. If one heel always wears down on the inside or outside, you definitely have a problem in structural balance.

7) Remove the incessant stress of poor posture habits. Check yourself and follow directions in this book for correction. Consult a professional to analyze your posture. Once you learn where the problem exists, you can put your body into a new and painless alignment.

FOCUS ON THE BIG PICTURE

Are you discovering there's more to backache, more to the body, than you originally thought? Well, don't be discouraged. All the bones, muscles, joints, ligaments, nerves and blood vessels you've been reading about will soon make sense and you'll see the big picture.

The more you know about yourself, the better patient you can become. The better patient you are, the more you can help your doctor . . . and that advantage you can't afford to miss.

The second dimension of the big picture means gaining confidence in your ability to make positive decisions.

Franz J. Ingelfinger, M.D., former editor of the New England Journal of Medicine, learned he had cancer and, because of his personal expertise in this field, was confused and worried. Finally a wise friend confided, "What you need is a doctor."

It was true.

Once he had made the decision that someone else should take care of his case, he found instant relief.

You are getting the big picture in becoming aware of the need for better posture, of using your body more efficiently, in sitting, standing and walking more erectly, in avoiding lifting and working in awkward or unnatural positions, in practicing stretching exercises to increase the distance you can move forward and backward, left and right.

If by now you realize you need a doctor to help, don't feel defeated. You may well be on the verge of victory.

In the next chapter, you will find enlightening—possibly even upsetting—information about the medical industry. At the very least, you'll learn how to get your dollar's worth at the doctor's office.

More importantly, you can find the way to locate a health professional who can take charge of your condition, dispel your concerns and help you toward recovery.

That's a promise.

CHAPTER 6
Don't Be Robbed At The
Medical Supermarket!

If you have a back or trick joint that goes out when and where you least expect it, you know too well the nightmarish experience: excruciating pain, gut-tightening anxiety, humiliation, and keen frustration that an otherwise perfect body is subject to a physical problem beyond your control.

Doubled over, grimacing, desperate, you try a nearby physician in your emergency, hoping against hope that he's a warm, kindly, caring family doctor. You are a generation too late.

The IBM computer efficiency of the office chills you. Suddenly you feel less like a patient and more like a "health consumer" in the medical supermarket system.

In your confused, vulnerable condition, you submit to a bewildering array of tests—most of which you suspect are not needed—all of which will cost more than you can afford.

Oh, how you wish you had been better prepared—less bewildered and more knowledgeable about your condition, about tests that are necessary, about the proper treatment required, about how to get your money's worth for services you are contracting.

Well, that's what this chapter is all about.

It's not intended to impugn anyone's reputation or to imply that any physician or institution intentionally seeks to rip you off—only to explain some of the little-known facts about modern medicine.

Many of the tests billed to you are ordered for legal

protection of the medical doctor, not necessarily to contribute to your treatment or over-all health.

Like you, the patient, the insurance industry has had to adapt to the requirements of today's medicine. Previously, a policy holder was required to be hospitalized before charges for a diagnostic exam would be covered. Now insurance firms see the economic futility of placing this obstacle before the doctor/patient relationship. The physician would merely hospitalize the patient for economic reasons, not a biological need.

While this may be considered humane, it does point out the crazy patchwork construction of the so-called health care industry. Even this terminology is weird. A person buys "health" insurance, which deals only with ill-health or infirmity. You can't buy health with it. It only pays off when sickness occurs.

You enter the "health" care system only when you're sick, not to build good health. And the whole complicated complex is regulated by the Health System Agency, a federal organization concerned with hospitals which want permission to add more beds or expensive equipment.

Whatever concern there may be for the community's health or state of wellness escapes detection.

So far as health insurance is concerned, be sure you're getting everything promised in large and small type. If the doctor doesn't get paid according to promises made by the insurance salesman or his colorful brochures, complain first to your insurance company or the brokerage firm which sold you the policy. If you don't get satisfaction there, write to the Insurance Commissioner of your state. Specifically describe your complaint. Your voice will be heard along with those of others who may receive fewer benefits than promised.

Many states have an insurance equality law. This provides that your policy must pay for services of the doctor of your choice, when this doctor uses the same procedures a doctor of another discipline would utilize.

Just as you can get your full money's worth out of insurance if you are prepared, you can do the same with the doctor. Anticipate an emergency and know everything possible about your bad back.

It pays to understand your insurance policy before an emergency. It also pays to be familiar with your doctor before your time of desperate need. Anticipate an emergency. Prepare for it by knowing everything possible about your doctor's treatment methods and procedures and, particularly, about your bad back.

Understanding your condition helps you determine within reasonable guidelines if your immediate problem is a true emergency and whether or not you can wait for treatment during the doctor's office hours without additional physical damage.

Part of your preparation for an emergency should be a written explanation of your physical impairment by a doctor. This will guide you to the proper action should an unexpected, acute incident occur. It will do three important things for emergency hospital personnel: offer critical input, the name, address and phone number of your doctor so that they can contact him, and help avoid duplication of examination procedures.

Be alert to several additional costs with which you can be hit in hospital emergency care: (1) X-rays (which probably exist already but may not be available during an emergency exam); (2) An examination which focuses on severity of the immediate condition—not of long-range, corrective diagnostic quality; (3) Lab tests for immediate purposes—not for a general assessment of your system; (4) Emergency room facilities—anywhere from $35 to $50; (5) Specialist care. (The emergency staff is not usually skilled in structural problems and will often advise calling in an orthopedic specialist or neurologist, which will add another $50 to $100 on to your bill); (6) Hospitalization for observation and medication is a better than 50-50 possibility. (Bed-rest at home may be more relaxing and beneficial); (7) Short-term use of braces, neck-collars or strapping. (This is often a duplication of devices you may already have at home). (8) Duplication and possible undesirable effects of medication.

Take the sting out of emergencies with foresight: 1) Have a written diagnosis and X-ray report from your doctor (this is your right) 2) Understand your problem 3) Don't allow your pain to override sound judgment.

Another way to squander good dollars is on bad advice.

Talking with too many "experts" about your condition can be hazardous to your health. Find one source for guidance. Welcome the concern of others who may be equally capable, but remember that too many opinions can add to your confusion and feelings of insecurity.

Any doctor can be guilty of giving good advice which turns out badly. I know. It happened to me recently with chilling impact. I advised an overweight patient to leave her car at the far end of the parking lot when shopping. The extra exercise would benefit her problem.

An hour after leaving my office, I received a phone call reporting that she had been mugged, her purse stolen. I learned from this experience that the police advise against this practice, urging people to park nearer stores and under lights.

Despite this unfortunate incident, I maintain that it is seldom wise to second guess your doctor, attorney or

CPA. However, you are better equipped to make judgments when you are fully briefed with the facts about your condition.

Being uninformed permits you to be wide open and vulnerable to remedies and treatment which act on symptoms, rather than the underlying cause of your problem. Believe me, this is the most expensive type of care that you can buy.

Not only does symptom-treatment cost a fortune, it prolongs your total recovery. When you overcome the basic problem, you eliminate the burdensome annoyance of symptoms, and the aching need to relieve them.

On the other hand, don't expect your doctor always to be infallible. He's not. No one is. Doctors are mortal, subject to human traits of prejudice, arrogance and common short-sightedness.

Among members of the healing arts, the most respected are those who admit they don't know everything. Every decade and every era in history bears this out, because what is gospel yesterday can be scorned today.

Physicians deal in temporary states of knowledge. "From what we know today . . ." is—or should be—the usual preface when presenting a diagnosis. Because tomorrow we may learn more about you, and that could change our original viewpoint.

One bit of advice not subject to change is that the least costly route to ending backache is through having a physical exam by someone skilled in correcting spinal and structural problems.

The more the consultation doctor knows about you and the history of your complaint, the better prepared he is to help. It is wise to supply the following information in advance of your appointment:

1. A written summary of your entire medical history.

2. X-rays.

3. Prior medical reports.

4. Your objective—what specific results you expect from the examination.

5. State whether or not you wish a written report on your examination and what purpose this will serve. (A narrative medical report fee ranges from $50 to $150).

RECOGNIZE WHICH DOCTOR IS YOUR "MR. RIGHT"

It is hard to believe in a doctor who doesn't believe in you and your physical complaint. Just what does that mean? Simply this: there's a tendency on all levels of society to discount the syndrome of backache. Some doctors are the biggest discounters.

Nobody, it seems, is interested in your complaint, and most of the people you complain to don't even believe you hurt. That's a fact.

However, if you could lie down and bleed, then everyone would be concerned and convinced that you actually suffer pain. But a back pain—forget it!

Obviously, if your doctor thinks your back pain is all in your head, you need another doctor. Fortunately there are doctors who specialize in back problems, individuals who know they are real. These practitioners may not necessarily look like the Hollywood stereotype of a physician. In fact, they may even be fairly rumpled in appearance, because they are bending, stooping, manipulating—working hard physically to relieve patients of their complaints.

Don't look for surface things. Find the doctor who will devote all the time and attention necessary to correct your condition.

Such a doctor is skilled in managing muscle and skeletal disorders, not limiting his practice to emergency care for broken bones. Favoring this treatment doesn't mean that you need to oppose all other types. Everything has its therapeutic place. What you need is a doctor who fits into place for you, your ailment and your ability to pay. Empathy is superior to sympathy for you.

IT'S YOUR BODY. DON'T LET OTHERS ABUSE IT

Do you realize that poor treatment may be more damaging to your body than no treatment at all? This is a documented fact. I have seen this in patients who have come to me. So have my many colleagues in chiropractic.

Some medical doctors in instances of birth defects and unusual disabilities due to severe trauma insist that lifetime treatment is necessary. Perhaps it is. Yet even in such cases, I have seen a measure of improvement through exercises presented in this book. These exercises have minimized or even eliminated the need for constant treatment.

In searching for the right doctor for you, there are two classifications to avoid or quit:

1. *The practitioner who constantly treats without positive results.* If you have been seeing a doctor regularly for one or more years and your condition is not markedly improved, chances are you've been taken. Get an opinion or two. Even try a different kind of treatment. Ask pointed questions, like: "Why does this condition persist?" Don't settle for double-talk. Get a specific answer.

2. *The doctor who prescribes medication which fails to*

correct your condition. If medication is the only prescribed form of care, face the distasteful fact that you are not overcoming your handicap. You are getting worse, more fixed. Even worse, you may have become drug-dependent and in more serious distress.

Receiving repeated injections of pain-relieving drugs or steriods can greatly damage and upset the function of your metabolic system. Examine the situation frankly. Are your hard-earned dollars going for relief of symptoms or for correction?

Does cortisone have the ability to correct a defect in your posture? Or, does it prolong the recognition of your true, over-riding problem?

Has your present treatment helped you at all? If not, why not? Is a total cure for your problem in sight? If the answer is "no," you are doing more for your doctor than he is for you.

If ligamentous damage has weakened the ability of a joint to maintain its normal alignment, you may benefit from life time care—however, treatment restores normalcy, it does not put off the day of reckoning, as would pain-deadening pills.

Few back problems should be expected to correct themselves without professional or self-help. What occurs is the muscle imbalance or bony misalignment encourages progressive structural compensation...you're trading one problem for another. Don't abuse the only body you'll ever have with neglect or with an unsatisfactory mode of therapy. Utilize your options for maximum relief.

THIRTEEN WAYS TO SAVE MONEY IN THE DOCTOR'S OFFICE

Backache is not only chronically painful physically ... it has the potential of being painful financially. You can save money spent in the doctor's office by following these

13 hints from my experience, those of health profession-als and consumer affairs authorities:

1. Always remember that a doctor needs full informa-tion about you and your condition. Prepare a brief but complete chronological medical history for him or her. If the doctor has to spend a great deal of time interview-ing you, his fee is often higher.

2. Follow directions honestly. If you disregard specific instructions, how can you measure benefits of your care?

3. If you disagree with advice given, voice your specific objection. Come to an agreeable compromise. Go else-where if you are being constantly challenged and feel uncomfortable.

4. Ask questions which provoke information rather than hostility. You can alienate yourself to the point of receiving non-caring attention.

5. Make sure that your doctor will willingly send your X-rays to another doctor of your choosing. If he won't, he is not the kind of doctor to deal with.

6. When you start with a new doctor, always provide him with a list of all substances which you are taking— also their potency.

7. Avoid what seem to be far-out health procedures. These may or may not be effective for certain ailments, but mechanical problems are usually not in this classifi-cation.

8. Don't go "doctor-shopping." This costs a lot and produces little. Each new physician will duplicate examinations. These won't contribute to your well-being. You already know you have a bad back. Your doctor's examination should be complete and lead to eventual correction of your problem, not to another referral.

9. Visit your doctor regularly. A treatment program

is usually more effective if observation and feedback can be used to correct your regime to your specific condition.

10. Ask the doctor if you may prepay costs for visits to save bookkeeping fees.

11. Be sensitive to when you are referred to another doctor simply because your doctor is not obtaining satisfactory results. This may be a device to end your association. You are the one who picks up the tab. A consultation with a specialist in another area of the body is not objectionable—frequently desirable—if it has been done to increase *your* doctor's chance of finding the proper solution to your problem.

12. Try the barter system if you're faced with a long-term recovery program which taxes your financial resources. Perhaps you can trade-out your services, or products, for the health care needed.

13. Talk with a knowledgeable pharmacist about generic substances. It is possible to buy aspirin—acetosalycic acid—at less cost than a "Brand Name" without sacrificing either quality or effectiveness.

CONTROL YOUR MEDICAL DESTINY— IT CAN BE FUN

Being in control of your life—your emotions, your physical well-being and your environment means living the way you want, the healthy way you should.

Being repressed, stuffed back inside your cage, can precipitate more than backache . . . sooner or later, you overflow with activity which even you recognize as being wild, senseless and totally unproductive of accomplishing your life's goals.

Relate this to stress, if you will, but in my experience

151

it appears more like failure to assert one's self, an attitude of defeat and submissiveness without relief. Once you give in, you are granting permission for the other party to continue taking advantage of you. You're putting up an umbrella of acceptance ... you're saying, "Ok, give it to me, I'll take it."

Where does it lead, this super-submissiveness? To a backache, that's where. All the repressed frustration, guilt and anger works its way out of your body through the joints, and, you know this hurts! You're a nice person with a bad back.

Mrs. G. was one of my patients who turned this scenario around.

It had been a month of appointments and cancellations before Mrs. G. finally arrived for her first visit.

"You must think I'm pretty strange, Dr. Lindsey," she said. "The truth is I haven't left my bedroom for three months . . . I've been afraid to leave the house. It took a week to get enough courage to call for an appointment, and three more to keep it."

Obviously Mrs. G., overweight and figidty, continually curling a loop of hair around a finger, was suffering a condition of regression. She had almost totally withdrawn from society.

Fortunately, with diet, nutritional counseling and correction of her back problem Mrs. G. responded swiftly and regained control over situations which were headed beyond her ability to cope.

"Would you believe I went bowling with my husband last night—and without a backache?"

Mrs. G. credited much of her recovery to our discussions which explained how the body works and simple explanation of basic anatomy. The sparkle of her eyes revealed how grateful she was to learn her pain was generated by pressure on a nerve in the upper back, not a terminal growth. Mrs. G. expressed a deep fear of cancer, but this couldn't match the confidence she gained from learning how the bones, muscles, nerves and blood vessels worked. She overwhelmed her fear with knowledge. Mrs. G. managed to regain control over her life.

If you experience foolish fears—which are not foolish at all—or obsessions, talk with your doctor. Gain the understanding of your body—you are gaining much from Bye Bye Backache—to put yourself in control of your medical destiny. You'll find it far more fun than the dread fear of the unknown. Knowing more about your body functions will make the "it could happen" less likely to happen . . . it could even make the possible impossible.

You'll learn how body chemical reactions can help a backache, or hurt one, in the next chapter which deals with nutrition and the need to supply all the tissues and brain with cell rebuilding substances.

CHAPTER 7
Nutritional Hints That Ease
Back Pain

Your common question, "Will changing my diet ease the pain in my back," does not have a common answer. But, somewhere in this chapter you will discover clues to solve your problem—relief from back and joint pain. The key is improved nutrition.

Since you react differently to food than anyone else— in your metabolism, digestion, absorption and assimilation—your total nutrient requirements are exclusive to your body. It's not a matter of personal taste, say of vanilla flavor over strawberry. Ice-cream may set well with you while it gives another person hives.

There is one uncomplicated rule to follow for good nutrition: *Nourish the individual cell.*

This rule applies to everyone, health food "nut" to junk-food junky. It's universal and crosses all boundaries of race, religion, ethnic/culture, environment, color, sex or age. The nutritional requirements of the human cell is identical in all peoples.

During my practice years I have found few, if any, patients who were not improved through nutritional counseling whether their back and joint problem resulted from birth defects, accidents, strain or arthritis. Seldom have I read a nutrition textbook that did not present evidence of world-wide protein, calcium, and vitamin C deficiencies.

What about the calcium intake of the inhabitants of impoverished areas of the globe? No, they don't take a convenient pill available to Americans and Europeans,

154

they supply this necessary mineral through diet—eating bone and cartilage. Calcium is recognized as an important nutritional problem in China, even though their cookery furnishes a large amount of the bone calcium which is not generally utilized in American households. Natives of the Arctic and some parts of Asia also consume bone and cartilage, while the turbid drinking water of Africa, plus the eating of coarse leaves and nuts, provides a dietary source of calcium and other minerals.

You can imagine how eating habits differ from country to country, but the basic requirement to sustain life is identical: *nourishment of the human cell.*

Diet—choosing which foods to eat—is a popular subject for discussion between the modern doctor and his patient. I've talked with many patients and doctors about diet and conclude there are three kinds of people

1) People who could care less about the consequences of what they eat. Their philosophy is: "If it was good enough for Pappy, it's good enough for me."

2) People who fool around with food. They constantly try "the latest" diet reported in the National Inquirer, Reader's Digest or in the weekly Food Section of the local newspaper. They seldom stick to the diet or remain loyal to the author by attempting to learn more about his or her program.

3) People who are truly interested in food as a source of body fuel and energy. They experiment widely and do adopt good eating habits. These people may be further subdivided into two groups: A) Those content merely to use trial-and-error and B) those who continue to read and study about nutrition to find the reasons behind the effects of feeling better, and, subsequently, relief of con-

stant muscle and joint pain or overcoming a physical handicap.

Everyone plagued with chronic muscle pain or stiffness, bone ache or limiting physical disorder benefits from gaining a working understanding of how the food you eat affects the tissues of your body. The health of tissues and organs is involved, and, in backache, even a little bit of knowledge is helpful.

Jerry, a 32-year old carpenter, was a skeptical person who fell into the No. 1 category above. "How can my diet have anything to do with my back pain?" he wanted to know.

While he was aware he was entering a "burn-out" phase in his occupation after twelve hard years hammering long nails into 2x4 studs, Jerry was tough to convince that an analysis of his hair might provide insight into his problem. He was without belief—but was willing to try anything.

The answer to Jerry's question, "What's my hair got to do with a stiff back?" arrived in a computer readout listing the mineral levels found in Jerry's hair analysis.

"Your calcium and phospherous is far out of balance and you're extremely low in iodine."

Jerry admitted he never drank milk, hated salads ("rabbit food") and sweated heavily and easily.

Taking a nutritional supplement of magnesium, phospherus-free calcium, vitamins D and C, eating more green, leafy vegetables and a protein cocktail three times daily put Jerry on the happier side of life . . . he was no longer stiff in the morning. He had reversed his condition of fibrositis, a form of arthritis which affects the connective tissues making them stiff, inflexible and constantly ache.

156

Becoming familiar with the dynamics of nutrition—the processes of digestion, absorption and elimination—relieves stress on sensitive tissues aggravated by eating the wrong foods.

Drinking orange juice can cause pain in the joints of an arthritic. Why?

A three-day distilled water fast fortified with vitamins and minerals, can ease the pain traveling from joint-to-joint in an arthritic patient. Why?

The answers to these questions revolve around the chemistry taking place in your body—in the liver, kidneys and individual tissues by allowing nutrients to enter the cell or blocking them out. The specific answer may lie in your acid/base balance, which is influenced by a dietary intake of protein or carbohydrates and fats.

The healing aspects of diet concerns the length of time you have been violating Nature's laws by over-eating, under-eating, unbalancing the nutritional needs of your body by neglecting certain important foods while pandering to exotic tastes of sugar, coffee and tea or alcohol. The damage of long-term habits may affect the very organs and systems now needed to reverse the ill effects you experience, the woe-begotten rewards of unfortunate dietary habit patterns.

Body chemistry involves more than sitting down to a meal and eating . . . it concerns every function occuring in your body, 24-hours a day, every day of your life. Eating and drinking, these are the most significant acts you perform in relation to your total health, certainly to tissues crying for help in your back and joints.

To grasp the impact of the nutrition-pain relationship, imagine how just one microscopic enzyme system alone can be involved in life-sustaining chemical reactions in

157

your body—and, it is estimated there are more than 80,000 enzyme systems circulating—or waiting to be manufactured by cells in your body.

Dr. Kurt Donsbach tells in *Preventive Organic Medicine* (Keats, New Canaan, Conn.) how getting out of step internally can hurt you. If even one tiny enzyme fails to perform its normal assignment in the digestive process, you can experience pain—the secondary pain of tissue irritation produced from toxic (incomplete chemical breakdown) products.

You understand many of the reasons for a backache from the physical concept . . . you must follow physical rules to avoid pain. Bending suddenly without preparing the muscles can cause back strain; lifting incorrectly will strain back muscles and ligaments; slouching, sleeping on a sagging mattress, or driving long distances without proper back support—these also cause backache.

But, what happens when you skip taking your daily ration of vitamin C? or calcium? or magnesium? Do you recognize the immediate symptoms this dietary oversight causes? Have you ever burped, aware of heartburn, and said, "Oops, I'm low on digestive enzymes?" Have you ever considered the sore at the corner of your mouth was due to lack of vitamin B complex? Or, the persistence of infection in a small wound and put the blame where it belongs on a deficiency of vitamin C?

You know moving in the wrong direction will produce an immediate symptom of pain. The source of this problem—the back—is instantly recognized. But, human biochemistry—the science of all the interactions occuring within the body—is still an intellectual infant compared to the knowledge of anatomy and *kinesiology* (study of movement). There is still much to learn about nutrition, it's not the exact science it should and will be in the future.

It is this exact uncertaintude which should lead everyone to err on the side of abundant nutrient intake, rather than accept indefinite standards imposed by institutional sources. Rely on your higher instincts, not the label on the cereal box.

A shortage of adequate nutrients—vitamins, minerals and enzymes—flowing in the bloodstream is difficult to detect compared to the dramatic jolt of a stabbing back pain. However, the insidious effects of nutritional deficiency can equal the backache if each of the individual symptoms are totalled: irritability, tiredness, mental confusion, lack of digestive well-being affecting appetite, digestion and elimination, muscle strength, cellular fluidity, harmonious endocrine activity, immune abilities, longevity, reproduction, sex drive and natural defense against invasive organisms. These are the fruits of good nutrition and an internal environment of biochemical balance.

If you're confused about nutrition and diet—no one can blame you—most people are.

Some doctors have a standard phrase for all questions about nutrition: "Just eat a balanced diet and you won't need vitamins and minerals."

Telling the overweight, underweight and nutritional wreck to eat a "balanced diet" is like telling an alcoholic not to drink; a smoker not to smoke; an insomniac to "go to sleep." This approach may keep the patient dependent upon the doctor, but it won't do much to imrove health through nutrition—it certainly won't help a backache.

159

But, again, who can blame the public for being confused.

One physician says, "You don't need vitamins and minerals, they are in the food you eat." While another doctor says, "You need vitamins and minerals, they are necessary for your health and processed foods do not contain the entire spectrum of elements required for optimum good health." Both are respected, learned practitioners. Which is right? Whose advise do you follow?

Unfortunately, *you* must make the decision.

Personally, I hope the simple logic of understanding the functions of these various essential substances—calcium, magnesium, phosphorus, vitamins D and C—will lead you to an intelligent choice between providing yourself a "safety factor" or the unnecessary risk of tissue starvation through deficiency.

THE CELL—NATURE'S BUILDING BLOCKS

You'll get more from your nutritional study by learning and understanding the individual cell. The body is composed of 100 trillion single cells, an identical group of which combine to create a tissue. When tissues combine, an organ is formed . . . an assembly of specific tissues performing specific functions.

Bones, muscles, ligaments, cartilage, these are tissues, a collection of identical cells. The liver, heart, stomach and the skin—the largest—are organs.

The strength and behavior of both these structures depend upon the individual strength of the single cell. Disease affects the cell, spreads to the tissues and to the organs. Cancer, for example, is an example of a cell gone wild . . . it proliferates crazily, without reason, without ceasing. A tumor is a collection of these crazy cells.

Therefore, good health—a sturdy back free of pain—relies upon the health and integrity of each dependent body—the cell—specifically to the cells forming connective tissue, largely associated with muscle, tendon and ligament pain.

"How can I help my backache with nutrition, a change in diet or by adding a few essential ingredients, such as vitamins, minerals and enzymes?"

Verworn. a renowned nutritional investigator, said; "It is to the cell that the study of every bodily function sooner or later drives us." So, let's examine what a cell is made of.

The bulk of a cell is composed of protoplasm (cytoplasm) "the stuff of life," which is the first cousin to the white of a raw egg, a water-loving gel or *colloid* (the Greek word for glue). Protoplasm is protein in substance. The essential known elements of a cell are: calcium, magnesium, potassium, water, fats and inorganic salts and enzymes.

The cellular wall, or membrane, is, in some parts, sieve-like, allowing the passage *in* of certain substances and the passage *out* of waste products. The cellular membrane is selective in its action (osmosis) and responds to stimulation from chemical messengers sent by the brain and members of the endocrine system, which releases hormones from the thyroid, ovaries, prostate, parathy-

161

roid, adrenals, pancreas, and pituitary glands. The cell floats in a watery medium which maintains a somewhat constant acid-alkaline media. When dietary intake influences the normal pH (acid-base balance) it disturbs the normal homeostasis of the cells and causes many unfavorable results. (Eating pickles causes acid formation, while eating soda crackers—sodium bicarbonate—causes an alkaline reaction. Carbohydrate intake produces alkalinity, while protein produces a more acid reaction in the body).

A live cell is distinguished from a dead cell in its ability to: 1) grow 2) reproduce and 3) metabolize.

Metabolism, the act of building up or tearing down (catabolic) processes of a chemical reaction—the changes which take place when you eat food, may be influenced by your diet. If hydrocholoric acid, required to digest protein (meat, fish, eggs, poultry, dairy products) is absent in the stomach, the digestion (metabolism) will not properly occur. This end-result will be formation of catabolites (toxins) and cause digestive upset . . . and muscle pain.

Toxic materials occur in muscle tissues when lactic acid (and pyruuvic acid) accumulate and are not burned off (oxidized) by exercise. You recognize when this action occurs—you get your "second" wind. Muscle cramps are symptoms of incomplete chemical reactions which require adequate calcium or oxygen to release the irritant responsible for the cramp.

Oxygen is required for metabolism. In fact, internal chemical exchanges (oxidation-reduction) fail to occur without sufficient oxygen.

You know a blaze can be extinguished by smothering it . . . without oxygen the fire goes out. In the body without oxygen life goes out—in about three minutes. Think of the chemical reactions in your body like a bucket brigade carrying oxygen to keep the blaze alive . . . if those buckets fail to move along the line, the structure is destroyed.

Vitamin C and E are both important properties since they act as oxygen-savers, anti-oxidents...they protect your tissue supply of oxygen, allowing changes in the nutritive processes between cells.

Accompanying what is being called a wave of "Patient Awareness"—doctors are on notice the public is growing smarter, more discriminating, more perceptive, intelligent and sophisticated in health matters (bless them!)—is a corresponding demand for knowledge about nutrition.

Many of your questions are very complex, many require answers built slowly, step-by-step, for thorough comprehension.

That's fine, but it's not always possible to satisfy your hunger during office hours, when the doctor is busy working on your ailing bones and muscles.

You have a couple of alternative solutions.

First, since there are more good doctors than bad ones, it's possible to schedule an appointment to talk nutrition, a counseling session. This may accomplish your objective more meaningfully than grabbing partial or unsatisfactory answers. And, you allow your doctor to share your new-found enthusiasm.

Secondly, take advantage of the world of books, especially the reference materials available at your library. An excellent source for a storehouse of general information is *Nutritional Almanac*, Nutrition Search, 706 Second Ave. South, Minneapolis, Minn. 55042. Adelle Davis' books—*Let's Eat Right, Let's Get Well, Let's Cook*

It Right, and *Let's Eat Right To Keep Fit*—allows you to explore the entire spectrum of food health. Health food stores offer wonderfully informative magazines: *Prevention, Let's LIVE* and *Healthways*, among others. Copious amounts of free literature, on every aspect of diet and nutrition, is available from state universities and from local, state and national government sources.

Right now—on your own—you're looking for a practical guide to end back pain, free your joints from stiffness, soften rigid muscle cramps and, generally, replace your tight body with the flexibility of more youthful days. This can be accomplished and nutrition can help you reach these goals.

Diet alone can't undo the existing damage of solidified joints, but, in conjunction with other indicated therapy, nutrition can speed your body to better times. Nutrition helps your body to heal itself. How? You already have the secret: Nourish the cells.

Every illness places special stress upon the body. Musculo-skeletal problems—even simple strains—are no exception to the basic rules of physiology. The damaged tissues, especially the connective tissues, need extra nutritional support. Furthermore, remedies are indicated for the digestive factors associated with back distress, such as the constipation associated with back pain and lack of normal intestinal muscular activity, excessive gas, lack of appetite and other metabolic disturbances, all influenced by dominance in your sympathetic branch of the autonomic nervous system.

A normal, healthy body requires basic substances— carbohydrates, fats, protein, vitamins, minerals, air and water—called nutrients. These ingredients undergo chemical changes within your body—the metabolic

164

processes—which are vital to support life. These are recognized as the ability to: 1) grow and repair cells 2) produce heat and energy and 3) help in regulating various body processes.

PROTEINS

With back distress your need for protein is increased to rebuild cells damaged by strains or injury from auto accidents, contact sports, excessive exercise and exertion, and disease or illness, which is destructive to cells and tissues.

Repairing damaged tissues is not the same as building muscles or being active in athletic competition. Excessive intake of protein, in any form, powder, pills or food, is not as effective as many budding competitors believe. In fact, unbalancing your diet to build bigger muscles can be harmful. It is advisable to obtain all the facts, which point to a balanced diet of protein, fat and carbohydrate, plus vitamin and mineral supplementation, as the most effective program to attain constant strength and physical balance.

One of the easier ways to increase your protein intake is with a protein cocktail: Mix 2 heaping teaspoons of powdered protein into a glass of milk, fruit juice or water and blend in 1 tablespoon of wheat germ, a raw egg and fruit (bananas are excellent for flavor). Drink one to three of these energy-bombs daily. (Powdered Protein is available at health food stores, drug stores and in many doctor's offices).

Protein is your most important source for nourishing goodness needed by muscles and blood, the brain and heart. All of the amino acids are required before a protein is effective, this includes: leucine, isoleucine, lysine, methionine, phenylalanine, threonine, tryptophane, valine and possibly, histidine and arginine. Amino acids are the smaller units of the protein molecule. Some foods may lack certain of the above essential amino acids, and can be made complete by combining with foods which contain the missing amino acids. An example is eating beans and corn to obtain all the essential amino acids. Macaroni and cheese is another food combination which complements each other in supplying amino acids.

VITAMINS

Vitamins are found in food. Only vitamin D, and some B vitamins which are synthesized by bacterial action in the intestine, is manufactured in the body. Chemically, they are designated as catalysts, they alter the speed of a chemical reaction without entering into it. Vitamins are divided into two main groups:
1) Water soluble (they dissolve in water): B complex, C and bioflavinoids.
2) Oil Soluble (they dissolve in fats and oils): A, D, E, and K (fatty acids are known as vitamin P).

Vitamins enter into the function of enzymic activity and they must be obtained daily from foods you eat. They are not stored, except for A and D, in the body.

Oil soluble vitamins:
Vitamin A

While vitamin A is important for healthy complexion

166

and eyesight, it also is beneficial for rebuilding damaged cells and maintaining resiliency in ligaments and other supporting structures surrounding bony joints. It possibly plays an important role in keeping a constant level of moisture in the *synovial sacs* (and the *bursae*), the lubricating fluid which keeps the joints oiled.

Foods high in vitamin A are fruits and vegetables, butter and certain fish.

Vitamin D

Vitamin D is important in backache due to its action which regulates the levels of calcium and phosphorus in the bloodstream. Without this vitamin, these minerals are not absorbed or utilized by the body.

While small amounts are contained in fish liver oils and bone meal, your requirements for vitamin D are supplied through the action of ultra-violet (sunlight) upon your skin, converting a form of cholesterol into vitamin D.

A deficiency of calcium leads to osteoporosis, a softening of bone caused by allowing the calcium, which is normally found in bone, to drain out into the bloodstream. Another effect of calcium deficiency is tetany, uncontrollable cramping of the muscles.

The flow of calcium between the bone and tissues is also influenced by the secretion of the hormone from a tiny gland located on either side of the thyroid gland in the Adam's apple area of the neck, the parathyroid gland, in harmony with vitamin D.

Pollution can affect your absorption of vitamin D due to the haze which shields out the ultra-violet rays of the sun, as can clouds, windows and clothing.

167

Vitamin E

Vitamin E plays a significant role in healing injury to back tissues since it interacts with the adrenal and pituitary glands. During stress there is an exceptional demand placed upon the adrenal gland. A vitamin E deficiency—or the upsetting influence of backache—can disrupt the existing harmony within your entire ductless gland system. Adrenal fatigue depresses the stabilizing effect of insulin upon blood sugar levels and predisposes to diabetes.

Vegetable oils, shortening and margarine, plus whole grains, eggs, organ meats and some fruits and vegetables are rich in vitamin E.

Vitamin E is beneficial to the health of vascular systems. Following injury, the damage to small vessels must be repaired to reestablish circulation of fresh blood and to drain the area of fluids which tend to accumulate.

As an anti-oxident, this vitamin is concerned with the aging processes and has been linked favorably with improved fertility.

Water-soluble vitamins:
Vitamin C

In order of importance, vitamin C ranks as the high-priest of connective tissues, the glistening, almost-transparant, thin layers of tissue surrounding muscles (facia and membranes) and nerves, ligaments, and tendons. Cartilage, the soft, resilient—but thick and tough—material which covers the ends of bone to prevent friction and allow joint movement, is also composed of connective tissue. It also forms the bulk of the strange material of

168

the intervertebral disc—a soft, semi-elastic, spongy—
a kind of rubbery-plastic substance—which separates
the bones from each other in the spinal column.

The principal function of Vitamin C is formation of col-
legen, the inter-cellular cement which binds body tissues
together. Ascorbic acid (vitamin C) is the basic ingredient of scar tissue. Problems in movement occur when
the inelastic scar tissue infiltrates healthy muscle and
ligamentous tissues. Like adhesions following surgery,
these spikes of tough tissue restrict normal back movement. Scarring the walls of blood vessels can have
damaging effects leading to constriction of vital parts of
the blood-vascular system.

A supplementation of iron is usually required following injury to replace lost blood. Vitamin C is necessary
for the proper absorption and assimilation of iron.

The classic symptom of vitamin C deficiency is bleed-
ing gums, however, it also is associated with swollen and
painful joints, especially in arthritic conditions.

Many arthritics cannot tolerate citrus juces. This
leads to a vitamin C deficiency, which, many investi-
gators believe, is the result of a metabolic-allergic condition, some form of perversion within the digestive apparatus tending to abort normal utilization of vitamin C,
which further interferes with absorption of calcium and
other important minerals.

In cases of generalized joint pain—referred by many
patients as "creeping arthritis"—a complete dietary
overhaul may be beneficial, especially tests to determine
levels of the important mineral ratios (calcium to phosphorus, etc.) A program based upon the results of your
tests should be undertaken to promote balance between
the hormonal/nutritional/nerve systems. While this

appears a gigantic step, it can be accomplished by replacing the foods causing your distress with foods which do not irritate your tissues.

Remember always that your body needs increase during times of stress, infection and other periods when you're out of tune. Vitamin C is more sensitive to changes in your internal and external environment and emotional equilibrium than any other substance.

This important contributor of your total health is found in fruits and vegetables.

Vitamin B (Complex)

Vitamin B is actually a family of members known as a complex and includes B-1, 2, 6, and 12, plus biotin, choline, folic acid, inositol, niacin, pantothenic acid, para-aminobenzoic acid (PABA), Pangamic acid and laetrile (B-17). The most common member of the complex is Thiamine, vitamin B-1.

The highest concentration of the B vitamins is found in heart, liver, kidneys, brain and skeletal muscles. The complex is indispensible to the chain reaction of functions occuring in the Central Nervous System. It is also vital to the enzymic action taking place in the digestive system, acting as a co-enzyme.

The principal site of activity involving the vitamin/enzyme relationship is the small intestine, where carbohydrates are converted into energy-producing glucose, a simple sugar. When the body demands energy, the liver converts glycogen—a stored form of glucose—into glucose, the fuel which turns our wheels and spells the difference between vigorous activity and sluggish health.

Indigestion, the undesirable partner of backache, results from the incomplete breakdown of carbohydrates due to vitamin B deficiency. Stated another way, your "normal" intake of vitamin B may be dangerously low during periods of stress or backache.

Food sources for the "B" complex are whole grains, organ meats, eggs, legumes and nuts.

The Minerals:
Calcium

Without question, the most important and abundant constituent of the human body is the mineral calcium. Calcium is deposited and remains stored in the bone, entering the bloodstream upon demand by the body. It assists in blood clotting and enters into a variety of chemical reactions necessary for the function of nerves and muscles, and in regulating the acid/base levels of the body fluids.

In addition to vitamin D and parathyroid secretion, normal absorption of calcium is dependent upon an equal proportion of the mineral phosphorus. Normally a ratio of two parts calcium to one part phosphorus exists in the bloodstream. This balance can be tilted in favor of phosphorus when calcium is not being properly absorbed, due to excessive intake of fat foods and oxalic acid, found in chocolate, spinach and rhubarb. Large amounts of the phytic acid, present in cereals and grains, may also inhibit calcium utilization in the body. Deficiency of vitamins A and C also can be factors of poor calcium absorption.

Calcium is crucial to the transmission of nerve impulses, and a below-normal level of circulating calcium results in muscle cramps, numbness, "night leg twitches," tingling sensations in the arms and legs resembling the eerie feeling of an extremity which has "gone to sleep." Osteomalacia, a calcium deficiency disease is recognized by brittleness and fragility in bones and is frequently related to the aging process. However, some authorities believe this condition results primarily from lack of protein intake, a common dietary fault of older people. The carbohydrate imbalance contributes to inadequate absorption and assimilation of calcium.

Dairy products, especially milk, is high in its calcium content. The soft bones of fish found in canned salmon and sardines is a rich source of bone calcium. The green leafy vegetables are a non-protein source of calcium.

Phosphorus

Every cell in the body contains phosphorus, a frequent substance required for many of the body's chemical reactions. It maintains a constant 2:1 ratio with calcium in the body.

Phosphorus is an important part of the cellular repair process, especially critical following injury or illness. It also exerts an active role in the utilization of carbohydrates, fats and proteins, the production of energy.

Without phosphorus the heart and muscles would have no ability to contract, and nerve impulses would not occur. It is dependent upon vitamin D and calcium for its absorption.

Since it functions largely in the production of bone—in association with calcium—it is related to bone ailments, such as fractures, osteomalacia, osteoporosis, rickets and stunted growth, as well as disorders of teeth

172

and gums.

Meat is a good source of phosphorus, and fish, legumes and dairy products are also rich in this vital mineral.

Magnesium

Another close companion of the calcium-phosphorus clanship is magnesium. Half the body's supply is combined with calcium and phosphorus in the bones, the remainder in red blood cells and other tissues. All these are concerned with backache.

Magnesium is concerned with the regulation of body temperature and, through its related functions with the body fluids, also has an influence upon constipation. A danger may exist when this mineral is taken over a long period of time since excessive levels can increase the elimination of calcium and phosphorus.

A higher intake of magnesium is indicated when you take a supplementation of protein, phosphorus and calcium.

Manganese

This mineral also functions as an essential element in the activation of many enzyme systems, in addition to its role in carbohydrate and fat production. It contributes to the formation of vitamin B-1 and is vital to development of normal skeletal bones.

Manganese is found in tea, wheat germ, seeds, meat and whole grains.

OSTEOPOROSIS

How serious is this condition? Reliable data shows that 40,000 of the 200,000 women who will break their hip this year will die.

Osteoporosis (thinning of bone) is characterized by degeneration of bone mass. It is not accompanied by symptoms. The first knowledge of this condition may come to light following an accidental injury to the back or hip joint.

Malabsorbtion of calcium may be a primary cause of this deficiency disease. While some controversy surrounds the amounts of calcium required to avoid bone loss, many authorities believe 1200 to 1500 mg. is required daily. Exercise tends to strengthen bone mass, but do so with caution since a weak spine can collapse due to calcium loss.

Summary:

While not all the elements have been covered, the principal vitamins and minerals concerned with backache, muscle problems and abnormal conditions affecting bone have been,

If you suspect a deficiency, consult a good source for nutritional information and have them recommend a formula suited to your particular needs.

Right now, you are generously prepared to enter the final chapter, the therapeutic phases designed to end your back pain. Get ready to say "Bye Bye Backache."

NUTRITIONAL SUMMARY

FOOD	=	NUTRITION	=	ABSORPTION	=	METABOLISM
1. Carbohydrate		1. Energy		Digestion:		Catabolism
2. Fat		2. Reproduce cells—Growth		1. Enzymes		1. End Products
3. Protein		3. Regulate temperature		2. Vitamins		2. Body Functions
4. Vitamins				3. Minerals		3. Excretion
5. Minerals				4. Glandular secretions		4. Blood Circulation
6. Water				5. Hormones		

CARBOHYDRATE (4 calories)

1. Sugars   Glucose
   a) Simple: Honey, fruit
   b) Double: Table sugar
   c) Starches: Require
      prolonged enzyme action
2. Glycogen

FATS (Lipids) (9)

1. Saturated—
   contains hydrogen
2. Unsaturated—
   No hydrogen
3. Essential
   Fatty Acids
   a) Animal sources

PROTEIN (4)

1. Animal sources (fish, meat
   poultry, dairy)
2. Legumes
3. Amino Acids:
   a) Essential
   b) Non-essential
4. Combinations of
   Amino Acid Foods

CHAPTER 8
How To Say "Bye Bye" To Backache

Consider this final chapter as a new beginning.

Use this information to turn your life around and free yourself from fear of pain in the back. You're prepared, you've covered the basics, the groundwork which has elevated you to this plateau. Now you're ready to do what countless others have done—adopt and practice the methods which can reverse your present patterns of backache.

What's holding you back? I hope it's not the expectation of something complicated, because complicated things seldom work. In my years of practice, I've found magic in simple things—little things you understand, tolerate and accomplish without a heavy burden of sacrifice—this is the miracle stuff . . . little things you will do everyday. Isn't it the wrong little things you've done over the years that contribute to your present condition? It's time to work yourself back to a painfree state.

What can stand in your way? The only obstacle keeping you from total success is any remaining doubt, confusion or misconceptions. It's your turn now to be affirmative. Take a giant step and put your belief where it benefits you the most, in yourself. Match what you believe with the consensus of professional opinions:

1) Accept the truth that something is wrong. Don't neglect a problem that could get worse, even beyond repair.

2) Try conservative care. Nothing is lost through an

early program of posture correction, improved body mechanics, strengthening weak muscle groups and correction of nutritional deficiencies.

3) The doctor doesn't heal your body, *you do.* The stronger your faith, the more forcefully you believe in your ability to get well, the more certain you can be to attain your health goals . . . freedom from backache.

4) Work with a competent doctor who understands your problem and is willing to devote his energy and interest in your behalf.

How can you be so sure these remedies will work for you? Because you're not too feeble, too old or too stubborn to want to get rid of a physical problem that only brings you distress. And, you're far too wise to ignore the logic that making a few changes in your present lifestyle is worth it—if it means getting rid of backache. The following cases illustrate the simplicity attached to the solution of your problem, the roots of spinal irritation.

"Dr. Lindsey, I took part in every event of our company picnic over the weekend and today I'm hurting all over .. even in muscles I never knew I had."

"Do you make house calls, Dr.? I was building a cement block fence this weekend and today I can't get out of bed."

"My back is killing me, Dr. Lindsey. All I did was lean over to pick up a spoon and I haven't been able to straighten up since . . . "

Sound familiar? These Monday morning office calls all have one thing in common: Back strain due to bending too far. Sound too simple? Examine the logic, the dynamics. In a back that's tight and muscle bound, loaded with toxic wastes and on the imbalanced brink of disaster due to constant irritation from bad posture

177

and faulty mechanics, a strain or sprain is the only logical outcome. Precipitated by over-exertion and excessive bending—regardless of whether you were enjoying it, working at it or it occurred simply as a breakdown due to intolerance—moving beyond the limits of your joint capabilities results in disaster to the muscles, blood vessels, ligaments, nerves, tendons and cartilage associated with the back: a strain or sprain.

Regardless of the diagnostic title applied to your backache—even if it resulted from a birth defect—the sequence of events leading to your present anatomical abnormalcy is—or has been—precipitated and aggravated by back sprain.

This is the cycle of events which lead to backache:
1. Beginning with an imbalanced body you progress to
2. muscle tightness (or weakness) in one side of the body, which causes
3. malalignment in the spinal column, which causes
4. pressure on the bone (vertebra) and spinal nerve, which causes
5. over-production in connective and fibrous tissue cells which causes
6. disturbance in calcium metabolism which causes
7. roughening at the ends of bone which causes
8. wearing away, cracks and breaks in the smooth cartilage at the joints which causes
9. the body to react by contracting muscles (splinting) which reduces the distance in joint movement which causes
10. ad infinitum . . . .

Backache—pure and simple—is the end of this line. You can avoid this chain of events by being looser, increasing the flexibility in muscles, ligaments and tendons.

You increase your ability to bend, stoop, squat, stand, sit and lie down comfortably, without fearing back pain, by practicing the series of body movements presented in this chapter.

Whoa! Do I hear things like "I hate to exercise"?

Perhaps you associate the word "exercise" with punishment, like an irate coach telling you to "take an extra lap around the field." Or, you're just "naturally" a non-exerciser. That's OK, because I'm not suggesting a total fitness program. I ask only that you do not consider body movement as another of life's irritations . . . it's like brushing your teeth, the benefits outweigh the few minutes necessary to complete the action.

Every movement you make is exercise, so why not move in ways that help you—not hurt you? The basic activity suggested here lessens your chances of back strain. These are stretching movements which lengthen the muscles and ligaments. When muscles are misused or unused, the cells tend to "bunch up," accumulate in tight little bundles. During a massage you may feel these knots, even a light touch produces painful sensations.

The following stretching movements restore youthful flexibility to the spine, muscles and ligaments. They increase your range-of-motion. These are general in character and suitable for everyone, however, they are not to be performed against your doctor's instructions. Obtain permission, if you are under a doctor's care.

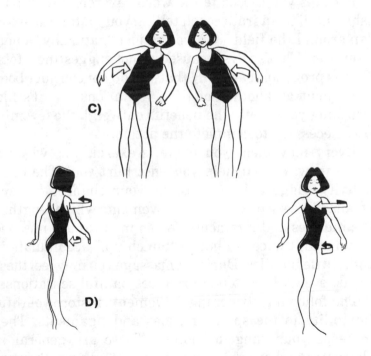

Fig. 55—Testing for range of motion in the lower back and torso involves A) forward (flexion), B) backward (extension), C) lateral and D) rotation movements. Record your first attempts at stretching and notice your progress as you practice these movements. Do not bend the knees in these movements. Do not try to move against resistance or pain.

180

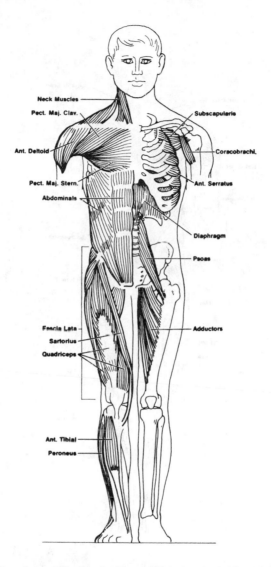

Neck Muscles

Pect. Maj. Clav.

Ant. Deltoid

Pect. Maj. Stern.

Abdominals

Subscapularis

Coracobrachi.

Ant. Serratus

Diaphragm

Psoas

Fascia Lata

Sartorius

Quadriceps

Adductors

Ant. Tibial

Peroneus

Fig. 56—Muscles of the body. In addition to stretching the muscles, the following movements in Chapter 8 stretch the ligaments and improve their elastic qualities. Disuse allows muscles to become short and knotty. Simple stretching movements tend to lengthen muscles, making them more supple and permit greater flexibility to the spinal joints, muscles and ligaments.

181

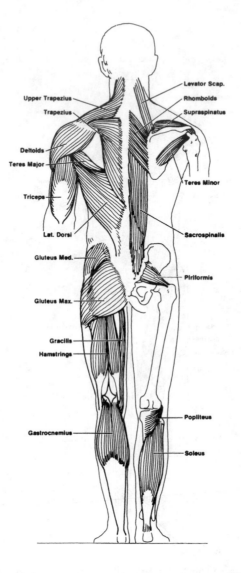

Levator Scap.
Rhomboids
Supraspinatus
Upper Trapezius
Trapezius
Deltoids
Teres Major
Teres Minor
Triceps
Lat. Dorsi
Sacrospinalis
Gluteus Med.
Piriformis
Gluteus Max.
Gracilis
Hamstrings
Popliteus
Gastrocnemius
Soleus

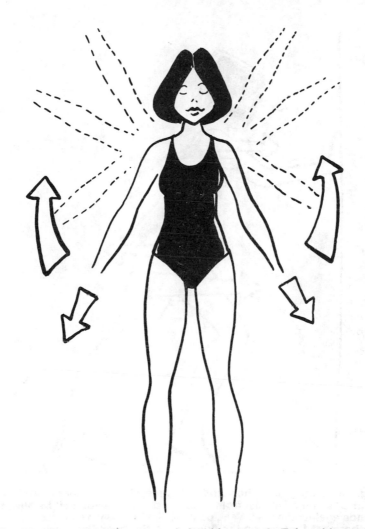

Fig. 57—Over-all trunk, arm and shoulder stretch. Take a big breath before starting and exhale as you push outward, hard as you can, with your arms. Lifting outward and upward until your arms are overhead. Exhale as you do this movement. You may need another breath when you reach the top, so keep your arms overhead while taking a breath and exhale as you lower your arms. Push on the downward excursion and exhale. One trip is sufficient to give you a warm glow over your shoulders and back. Try to push outward harder and farther each day you practice this movement.

183

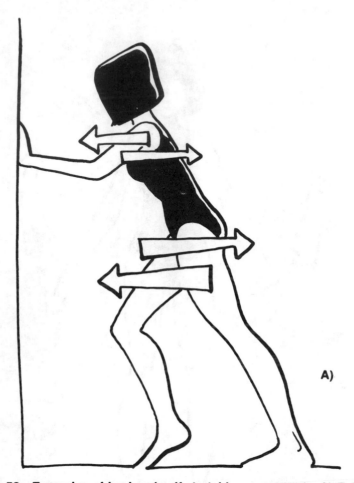

A)

Fig. 58—Examples of heel and calf stretching movements. A) Take
your position a few feet from a wall and balance yourself by placing
hands against the wall. Next, push against the wall while keeping the
farthermost foot flat on the floor. Keep the back flat. Pushing back
and forth, you will feel a pull on the heel cord and calf muscles. Try
to increase your distance from the wall as you progress with this
movement. B) Bouce up and down into a squat, keeping the back flat.
C) Stand on a 2 x 4 board and lower the heel. This stretches the heel
cord (Achilles tendon). D) With both hands against the wall push your
pelvis forward in short, quick movements. You should feel a pull in
the calf muscles. Repeat this movement several times daily and the
initial tenderness you experience will disappear.

184

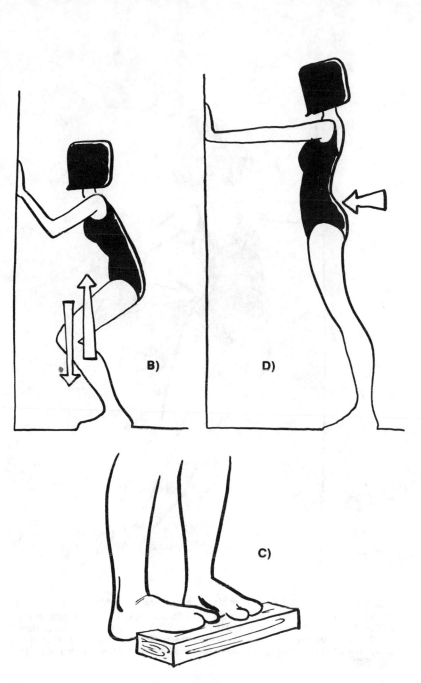

B)

D)

C)

185

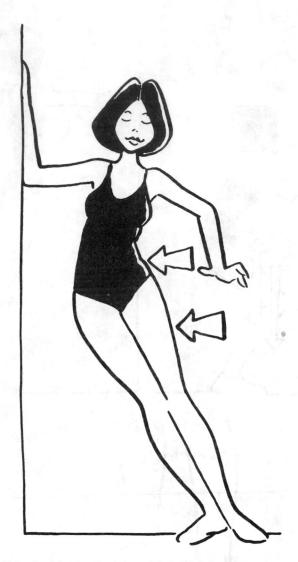

Fig. 59—Sideward body stretches for lateral flexibility and to over-come spinal curvature. Stand alongside a wall with feet together and allow the body to bend toward the wall. With a spinal curvature, bend on the side of the curve. This movement stretches the Tensor facia lata, the broad band of muscle located on the side of the hip (see Fig. 56).

186

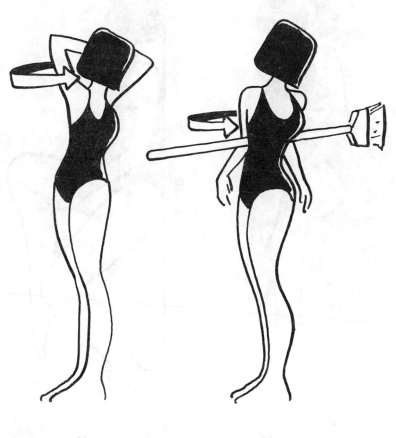

A) **B)**

Fig. 60—General twisting swings, right and left, to maximum limit of turn helps flexibility of trunk. This movement may also be tried with a broom, or golf club, held against the back while swinging back and forth with feet anchored. Do not turn your head while doing this movement, look straight ahead and notice how much further you move with each swing. Keep the back straight, eyes level and look straight ahead.

187

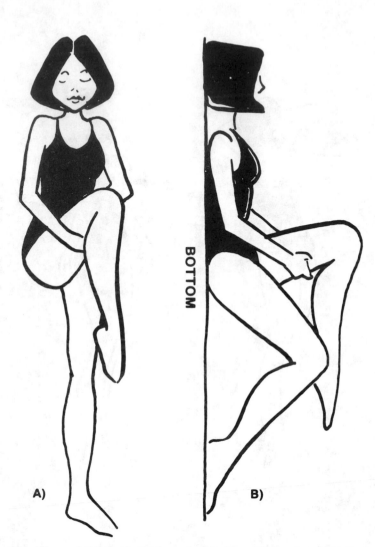

Fig. 61—Hip and thigh stretching, standing and lying down. A) Pull upward on one leg to stretch the thigh and hip. B) Lying down, the hip can be stretched by pulling the thigh toward the head. Allow the opposite leg to bend at the knee. Don't allow the low back to come up off the floor. C) A rocking stretch is accomplished by pulling both thighs toward the head and rocking. With each rocking motion pull a bit harder, attempting to get the knees as far upward on the chest as possible. Don't force. Greater mobility will come with practice.

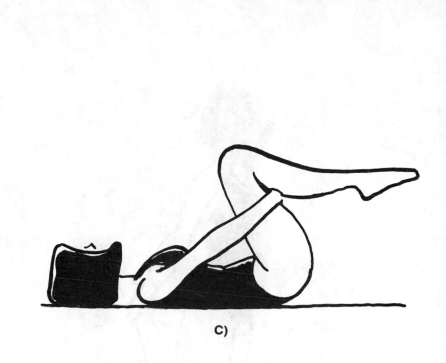

C)

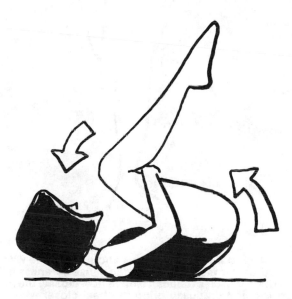

D)

189

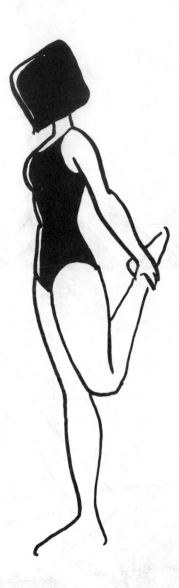

Fig. 62—Stretching the thigh muscles should be done with caution. Don't try to force this movement as it can cause soreness in the anterior (front) thigh muscles (quads). Notice how closely the heel comes to the buttock, and gradually bring the heel closer with repetition. Don't force this movement as it may also cause soreness in the knee.

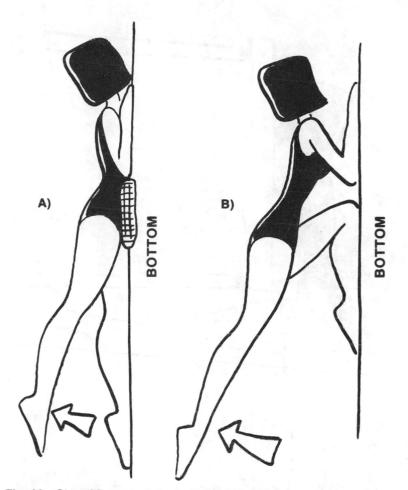

A)

B)

BOTTOM

BOTTOM

Fig. 63—Stretching movements to increase hip movement are done
lying face down on the floor. A) A pillow is placed under the abdomen
to keep the low back flat. Gently lift one leg upward while keeping the
stomach tucked into the pillow and the low back flat, without arching.
Don't attempt to overdo this exercise. B) Raise up on one knee and
repeat "A." Don't attempt to raise too far, allow gradual improvement.
C) Lying face down on a table with one foot anchored to the floor,
raise one leg upward from the floor. Keep the low back flat. You may
grip the table for additional support. In all three movements alternate
legs and notice if the height reached is identical. If one leg can be
raised higher, practice a few additional lifts with the weakened or
stiffer leg.

191

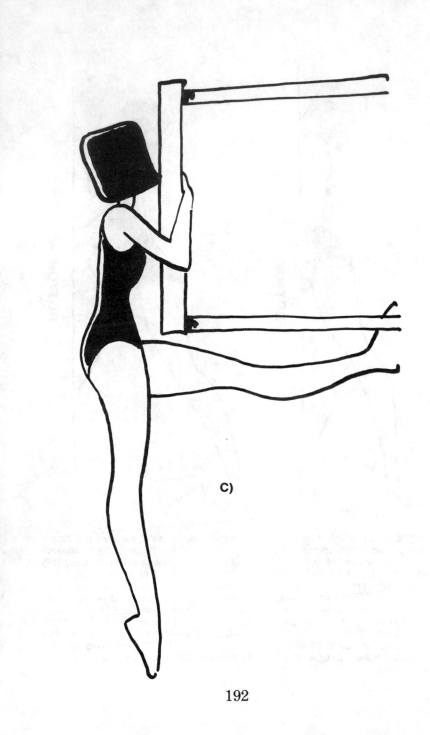

c)

192

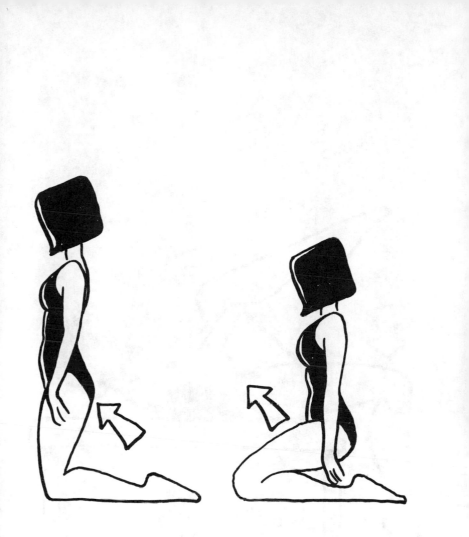

A)

Fig. 64—Kneeling exercises to increase hip flexibility. From a position of backward kneeling pull upward into an upright kneeling position. Keep the back straight, not bowed. If you have difficulty with this exercise, try strengthening the muscles with exercise B). Lying on a table, place a weight (sandbag or dumbell supported across the thigh) and pull the bent knee toward the chest. The other leg must remain level, as you do the exercise. Also, the low back must be kept flat, not arched. This movement relieves tightness in the area of the pubes and allows greater motion in the pelvic area.

193

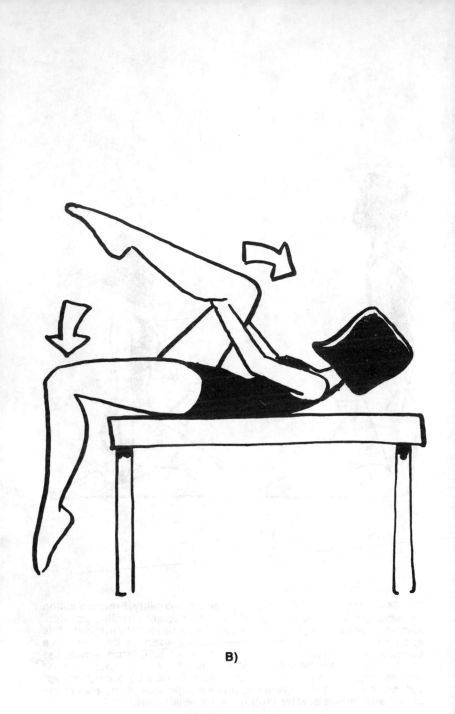

B)

194

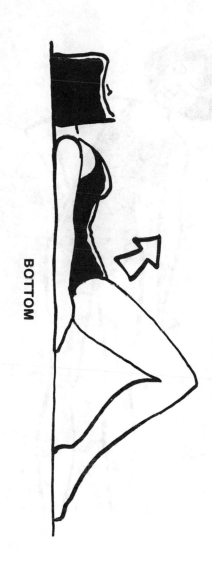

BOTTOM

Fig. 65—Low back strengthening exercise to overcome excessive curve in lumbar spine. Squeeze buttock muscles and pull upward from the pubes while keeping the low back flat on the floor.

195

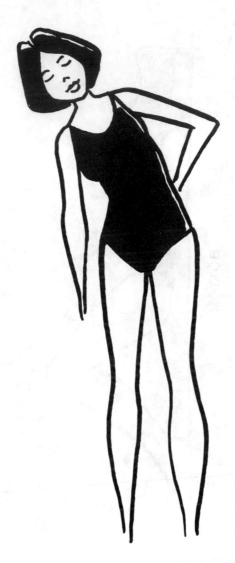

Fig. 66—Side stretches. Don't force while bending with the arm along-side the body far as possible, first to left, then to right. Mark where the fingertips reach their lowest point, and attempt to increase this distance daily. Do not force or bend the knees or the waist.

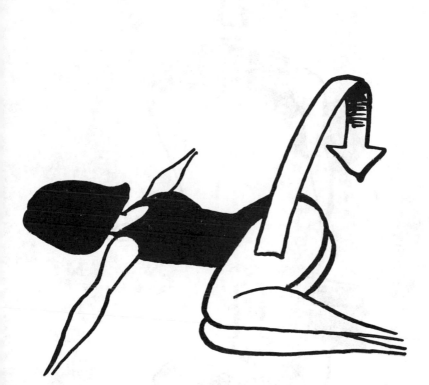

Fig. 67—Side-to-side hip swings. This allows the full spine to move as you swing the hips, with knees together, from right to left with slow, rhythmic movements. Don't try to move beyond any resistance or pain. If you encounter pain on one side, straighten both legs and bend the knee on the side opposite the pain. Pull this knee over to the painful side and press it downward to the floor, using your body as a lever to move in the direction opposite the pain.

197

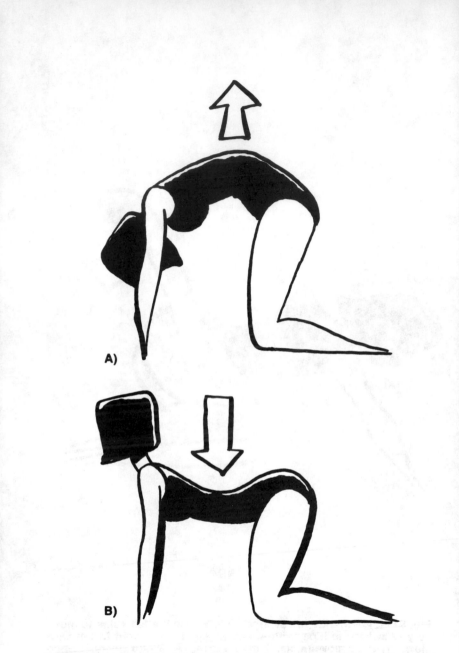

Fig. 68—Arching the back while on your hands and knees allows full mobility to spinal segments while B) allowing the torso to drop downward stretches the anterior (front) ligaments and muscles. This movement will relax a tired back.

198

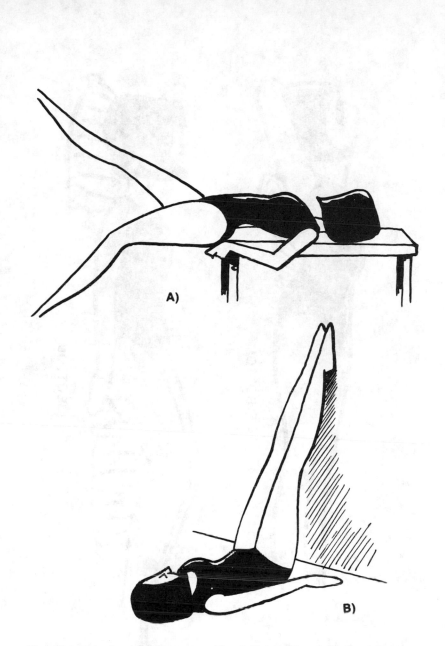

Fig. 69—Relaxing positions to off-set the strain of A) Oversitting. B) Overstanding. C) Working long hours at a desk. D) Over-exertion of the low back muscles, or strain. E) Relaxing position for relief of back muscle soreness.

199

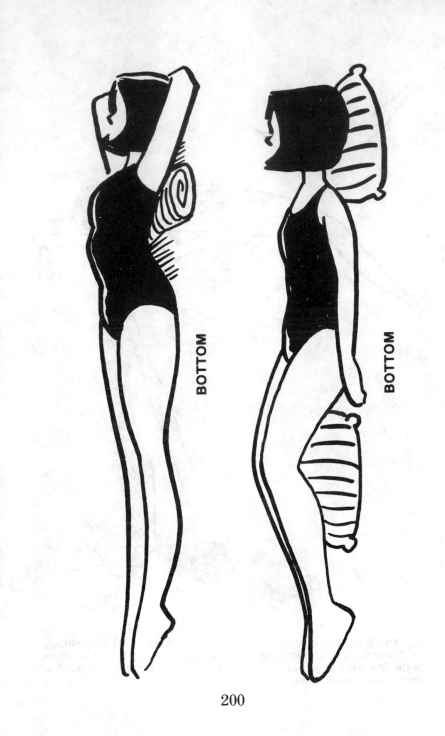

BOTTOM

BOTTOM

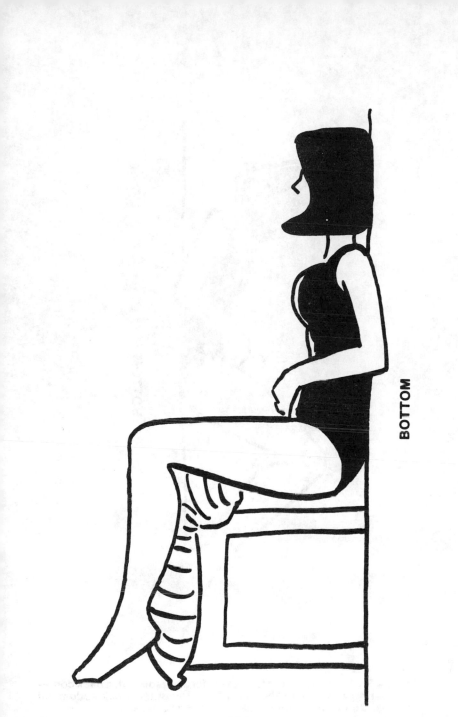

BOTTOM

201

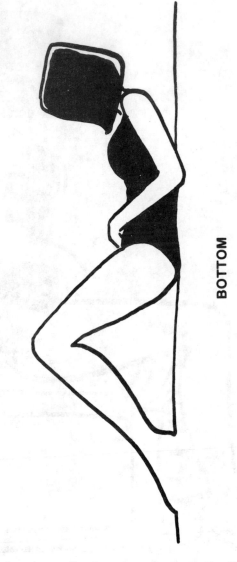

BOTTOM

Fig. 70—Push-ups are often too severe for a person with a back condition, therefore try these "head-ups" to strengthen weak abdominal muscles. Do not hold your breath for this exercise.

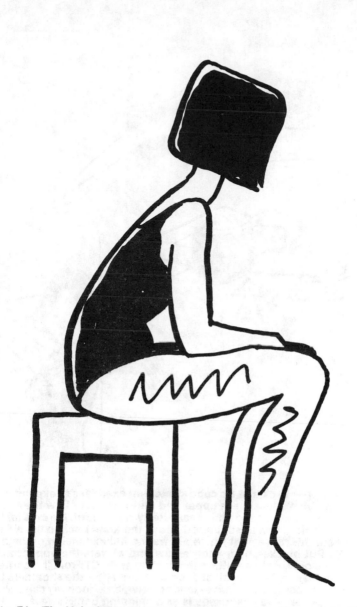

Fig. 71—The Valsalva maneuver is to be avoided during exercise. This movement occurs when the breath is held during exertion or resistance. The effect causes a negative downward pressure, causing pain in the inter-vertebral disc, rectal area. Increase bowel movements with natural methods, using fruit juices or bran to eliminate the need for force to evacuate the bowels.

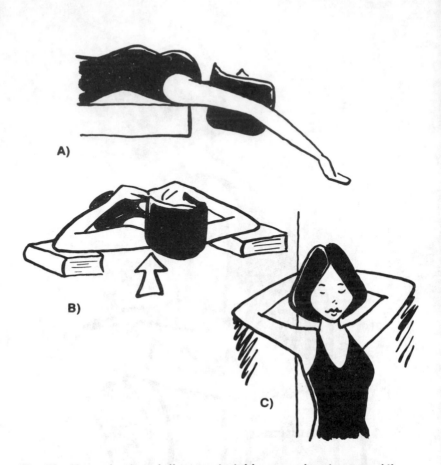

Fig. 72—Upper back and rib cage stretching exercises to expand the chest and relieve tension in upper and mid-back. A) Allow the arms to extend above the head and press slowly downward. Lie on a table or bed with the head unsupported. Move the arms back to the sides and repeat this movement which allows the full expansion of the rib cage. **B)** Put blocks under each elbow and elevate the upper back using arms only, not permitting the back to arch. **C)** From the corner of a room place elbows against each wall and allow the shoulders to drop into the corner. **D)** A bar extended between a doorway can serve many purposes. The best usage is as a chinning bar. However, with back problems it is best to merely hang, allowing your body weight to provide traction to the spine and joints. This operation allows blood to flow into the joint spaces of the back and relieves the pressure upon the intervertebral discs. Attempt to expand the chest while hanging. This excellent movement will accomplish much in just two to three minutes daily.

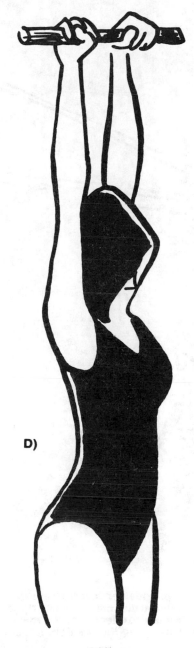

D)

205

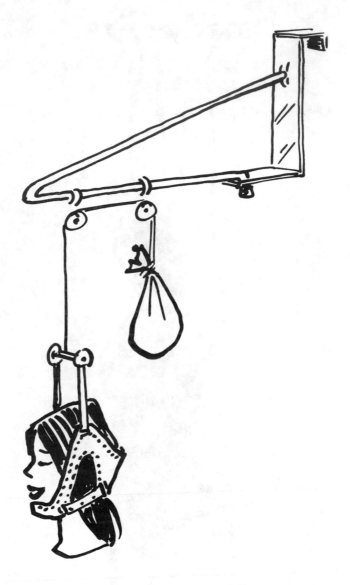

Fig. 73—A device to provide cervical traction to relieve tension and pressure upon the cervical disc can be easily rigged with the apparatus pictured here. This is also effective for headache relief. Sit straight in the chair while undergoing the traction, not slumped forward.

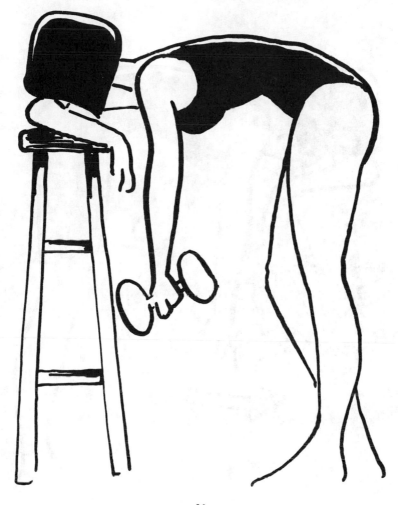

A)

Fig. 74—Traction to the shoulder joint is accomplished by resting the head against a table or stool and allowing the arm to swing freely, without undue muscular exertion. Holding a two to five pound dumbbell, book or can of food provides the weight necessary to open the joint and relieve pain.

207

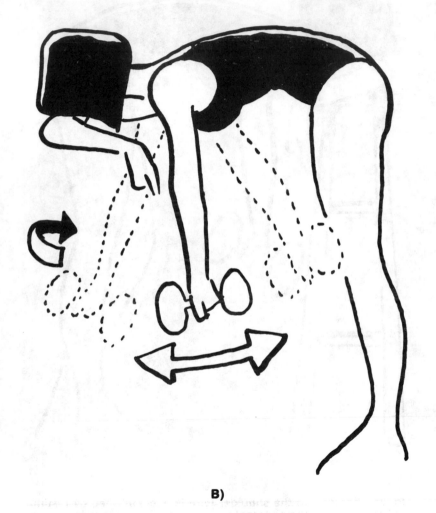

B)

208

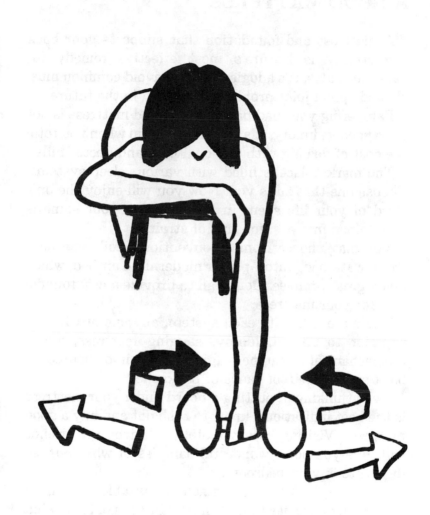

c)

PAMPER YOUR BAD BACK WITH A GOOD MATTRESS

A mattress and foundation that supports your back comfortably is Nature's most effective remedy for backache...also, it's a logical way to avoid common muscle and spinal joint problems, now and in the future.

Pampering your bad back with a good mattress is not an expensive luxury, it's a health bargain when you total the cost of dealing with personal pain and doctor bills.

The marketplace is filled with various sleep systems. Choose one that suits you. Now you will enjoy the one-third of your life spent in bed knowing your spine is maintained in a position free of strain.

You may choose from a conventional coil type mattress, waterbed, futon pad or modernized air bed, which holds great promise. Don't fail to provide a new foundation for your mattress.

There are merits to each system, any one of which is superior to an old, lumpy, sagging mattress, which biomechanical researchers agree is a common source for back strain, the root cause of backache.

Even thinking of putting a board under your mattress is the best indication I know to rush out and buy a good mattress. Visiting hotels, motels, relatives and friends will give you some wonderful samples of what *not* to duplicate in your bedroom.

Ask your doctor to recommend a suitable system for you. Experience has taught him what to avoid and what products provide corrective results. Also, he's aware his good work can be undone if you sleep eight hours with your spine in anatomically harmful positions.

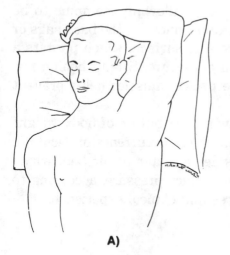
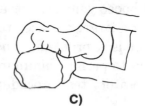

A)

C)

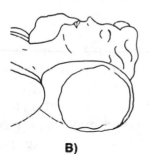

B)

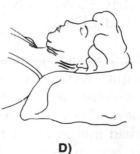

D)

Fig. 75—Proper and improper positions for restful sleep which do not produce back soreness. A) Sleeping with an arm overhead causes the arm to "go to sleep" and can awaken you by shutting off the circulation. B) and C) A round "Cervical" pillow prevents the neck from being strained and maintains the proper amount of curve in the neck during sleep. D) Hard, thick pillows, or sponge rubber pillows distort the normal curvature in the neck, causing soreness from strain.

211

The reason you awaken with a sore back is during sleep the back muscles relax, allowing the spine to be freed of muscle support. Consequently, the back sags or bows, especially on a too-soft surface, which permits a painful increase in spinal curvature. Strengthening low back, abdominal and the psosas muscles helps prevent this sag/pain cycle.

Choose your bed for even distribution of body weight over a larger surface area. If the occurrence of decubitis ulcer is a problem, consider a water or air bed, which tend to permit minimum surface pressure, according to laboratory test procedures and clinical experience.

MEDICAL NAMES FOR STRUCTURAL DISABILITIES

Understanding medical nomenclature allows some insight into the nature of your disability. Remember, conditions affecting the back are more frequently due to several causes, since, for example, inflammation may spread into neighboring tissues which may trigger reflex pain in more distant parts. Therefore, a diagnosis of strain may involve "radiculitis," the inflammation of a nerve root. Nevertheless, it may help you to better understand the doctor's evaluation of your case by sharing knowledge in widely used medical terminology.

RADICULITIS and other "-itis"

Radiculitis means inflammation of the root of a spinal nerve, especially where it exits from the opening between the back bones. A nerve can be inflamed by pressure caused by misplacement of the spinal bones in the neck (cervical), mid-back (thoracic-dorsal) or low back (lumbar). This condition may also be referred to as Cervical root compression syndrome, or cervical neuralgia. Radiculitis is also caused by injury, either of recent or past origin, postural strain, occupational and repetitive movements, whiplash-type injuries associated with rear-end accidents, athletic injuries (nose tackling), narrowing of the intervertebral foramen by the mineral deposits of arthritis, or due to a facet syndrome.

The suffix *"ITIS"* means inflammation. Therefore, you'll have no trouble indentifying: Tendon-itis, Myo (a prefix indicating muscle)-sitis, Fibro-sitis, Neur (nerve)-itis, Bur-sitis, etc.

The suffix *"ALGIA"* relates to pain. A muscle pain is myalgia, etc.

MISTAKES OF MOTHER NATURE:
SPONDYLOLYSIS AND SPONDYLOLISTHESIS

Unfortunately, mistakes do occur in the formation of the human frame. These are referred to as defects of birth, congenital anomalies or birth defects. The most obvious of these is scoliosis, an unnatural curving of the spine which occurs mainly in young, maturing girls (Fig. 76).

Spondylo (pertaining to a vertebra) plus lysis (to dissolve) is the dissolution of the posterior portion of a vertebra, usually in the area of the fifth lumbar.

Spondylolisthesis is a condition commonly found in the fifth lumbar area, but may occur elsewhere in the spine, affecting the ability of the vertebra to remain fixed in its normal position. The vertebra slides forward and downward on the sacrum due to a defect in the rear half of the vertebra. Repeated trauma is a contributing

213

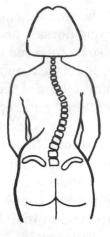

Fig. 76—"Idiopathic" scoliosis, a condition which affects the spine, mostly occuring in young girls.

factor in causing this defect to become symptomatic (Fig. 77).

A small patch of hair found over the sacrum may indicate underlying defěcts, such as *Spina Bifida Occulta* or *Spina Bifida Vera*, accompanied by a *meningocele* or *myelocele*, a tumerous growth in the sacral area.

SUPERNUMERY MEMBERS

Extra vertebra and ribs are not uncommon. They usually occur in the cervical area (Cervical rib) and lumbar spine. Having an extra lumbar vertebra (a sixth lumbar) may affect spinal balance and can cause frequent low back problems in individuals who perform manual labor.

SACRALIZATION

The lower portion of the lumbar spine is frequently the site of unusual bony formation. A *sacralization* is the attachment of the transverve process of a lumbar vertebra to the sacrum, making natural rhythmic movement in the fifth lumbar, pelvis and hip difficult, if not impossible. The basic problem associated with this

214

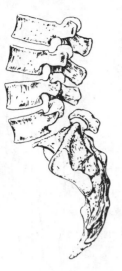

Fig. 77—Spondylolisthesis, a defect in formation of a vertebra which permits the segment to slide foreword.

immobilization is spinal imbalance and persistent muscular spasm and pain. By itself, sacralization is not considered a significant defect, but the effects generated by this overall imbalance causes back problems. Therefore, in all cases of structural abnormalcy consideration must be paid to establishing and maintaining ample balance to avoid consequences of compensation and painful adjustments related to a seemingly innocuous condition.

SCOLIOSIS

A lateral curving of the spine is called *scoliosis*. It can be either acquired or congenital in origin. The effects of "idiopathic" scoliosis is beyond the scope of this book, however, functional spinal curvature resulting from a short leg, muscular spasm, or muscular weakness on one side of the body can in most cases, be corrected with chiropractic adjustments to the spine and exercises which strengthen weak muscles.

215

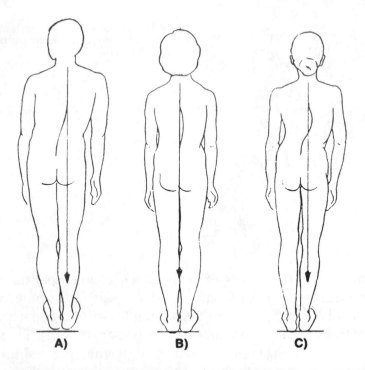

A)	B)	C)

Fig. 78—A "functional" spinal curve, which straightens when back is bent forward. This curving develops from strain, a short leg and incorrect posture.

LONG TERM EFFECTS OF STRAIN

What's the difference between a *strain* and a *sprain*? Both injuries hurt, can double you over and take you out of action. Both are related to a "catch" in your back or neck. They both involve abuse, overworking and overstretching tissues which support the back. You arrive at a strain or sprain as an aftermath of prolonged lifting of heavy objects, athletic activity, repeated twisting motions or from a rear-ender auto accident—yet, one

216

injury will go away without noticeable consequences while the other type may cripple you for life.

A *strain* is a case of muscular over-doing, too much exercise at home, at work or a recreational playground. With rest and liniment you recover quickly without after-effects.

A *sprain* is medically described as a wrenching type of injury which causes a partial tearing away of the damaged muscle, tendon or ligament from its normal attachment to a bony anchorage.

A *sprain* leaves some residual of permanent damage. For example, if you cut your skin it heals normally and it's over with. However, a cut in the skin leaves a scar which changes you. The scar becomes a residual of permanent damage. Even though the skin may now be stronger at the scarred area, your body—possibly your appearance—is not identical to what it was before cutting it.

Likewise, the healing which occurs following a sprain may procede normally, yet your body—and the damaged back tissues—will never be the same as before your injury.

Overstretching may leave a joint unstable, loose and without its former restraining abilities. It's like a rubber band that's been stretched too far, the elastic property is gone. An unstable joint, especially in the back, may need lifetime care due to its inability to maintain itself in alignment.

Frequently, a sprain injury, especially to the neck, may be described as "soft tissue damage," implying there is more than a single tissue involved. Although bones may not be broken, a forceful injury—a "whiplashing" rear-ender, for example—damages several tissues: muscle, longitudinal and capsular ligaments (which gives the joint its stability), the tiny blood vessels (the capillaries, arterioles and venules) which supply the spinal joints, tendons (extension of muscle tissue which attaches to bone), the fibrocartilagenous disc and the cartilage covering the surface at ends of bone where they join another bone to form a joint, the synovial sacs (possibly even the bursa), roots of spinal nerves, and, in time, reshaping of the injured bony segment itself. "Traumatic" arthritis is the result of severe strain.

That's a lot of damage just from a tap on the back or from bending over!

It proves a relationship between strain and Murphy's Law: Whatever can go wrong—will.

Examine Figure 79 (the spine). It brings the total picture—The Anatomy of a Backache-into focus.

Spinal vertebra are composed of a front portion (the body) and a back part (the neural arch). During early formation of the spine developmental errors may occur, causing an abnormal fusing or joining of the front and back portions of the vertebra (Spina Bifida is an example of improper fusing).

The rigid structure of the spine protects the spinal cord, which travels from the brain stem to the lower back, enclosed within a tube formed by the neural arch (the rear portion of the vertebra). Contents of the spinal cord constantly ripple back-and-forth in a flowing rhythm, and this movement can be affected by lack of flexibility in the pelvic area.

The 7-Cervical (neck) vertebra are the smallest, allowing the greatest trunk flexibility and motion to occur in the neck. The 12-Thoracic (dorsal—mid-back) vertebra also form a moveable joint with the twelve ribs, making

THE HUMAN SPINE

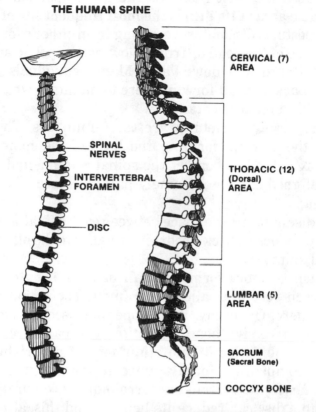

CERVICAL (7)
AREA

SPINAL
NERVES

INTERVERTEBRAL
FORAMEN

DISC

THORACIC (12)
(Dorsal)
AREA

LUMBAR (5)
AREA

SACRUM
(Sacral Bone)

COCCYX BONE

Fig. 79—The Human Spine. Individual segments of the spine are called vertebra. The 7 cervical are the smallest and allow the greatest range of motion. The 12 thoracic (dorsal) vertebrae also form a moveable joint with the twelve ribs, making this area the least moveable. The 5 Lumbar segments are the largest. The Fifth Lumbar sits atop the Sacral bone (the sacrum). Physiological curves in the lumbar (lower) area, mid-back (dorsal) and neck (cervical) regions permit an upright stance without strain. Muscle, tendons and ligaments concerned with balance attach (mostly to the transverse process) to the individual vertebra. There is a pad, a disc, between each vertebra. Spinal nerves exit from the foramen, an opening between the vertebrae. The facets, bony projections in the back portion of the vertebra, help maintain rigidity to the spine and limit lateral bending. The vertebrae form a tube, which contains the spinal cord traveling from the low back to the brain.

this area the least flexible. The lowest portion of the thoracic area (T10-T12) is the most frequent site of common postural discomfort resulting from either a forward carriage of the head or from allowing the pelvic area to tilt forward and downward. Many individuals allow their back to bend forward here to maintain what they "feel" is a balanced stance.

The largest vertebrae are the 5-Lumbars. They sit atop the sacrum, forming the base of the spine. The coccyx is the last bone of the spinal column, and when malaligned can be extremely painful, especially when sitting.

A disc occupies the space between each spinal segment and provides a shock absorbing quality to the otherwise rigid spine.

Each vertebra forms its half of the oblong opening between vertebra called a foramen. The spinal nerve exits here. Obviously, if this opening becomes smaller due to excessive bending action, encroachment by a facet, subluxation or malalignment of a vertebra, or from compressive force applied to the disc, the nerve becomes irritated from the surrounding pressure. Damage to a disc can reduce its heighth and this, also, narrows the space alloted for the unencumbered passage of the nerve from between two vertebrae.

The individual spinal joints are maintained in their normal alignment partially by the supporting action of the capsular ligaments—which bind around the joint—and the longitudinal ligaments, which attach and run parallel to the spine and by the facets.

Bony projections in the back portions of the vertebra—called facets—are an interlocking device which aid in maintaining structural alignment and limit lateral

220

movement of the trunk. Small sacs of fluid—the synovial sacs—found near the joints provide lubrication. Aging, disturbance in normal chemical reactions, inflammation and other damage to these sacs results in loss of fluid content and excessive friction at the joint. This may cause cracking noises within joint spaces.

The two wide bones on both sides of the pelvis are called the *Ilium* and connect with the upper leg bones *(Femur)* and to the sacral bone. This is the site of the popular "sacro-iliac slip," a gross misnomer since this joint doesn't "slip," it rotates obliquely, with one ilium going upward and backward, and the other appearing to move downward and foreward.

Ligaments supporting the female pelvis are stronger than are males, according to authorities. This quality probably relates to the child bearing function, when particular hormonal activity softens the binding cartilage and allows the pelvis to enlarge and widen. Following childbirth, this cartilage hardens again to its former strength. However, it is important to always examine the alignment of the pelvis no later than three months after delivery to detect any residual off-balance since this condition will result eventually in back strain and discomfort.

The spinal curves were described in an earlier chapter. Figure 80 shows how shifting the posture foreward or backward alters the normal spinal curves. The imbalance caused by allowing the pelvis to fall forward and downward changes the correct postural fulcrum, or axis, which normally counterbalances the constant gravitational pulling force on the erect body.

While treating an ex-professional football player for arthritis of the knees I asked him what he believed was the worst possible injury a player could have. He laughed loudly and said, "You're treating me for it, Doc."

221

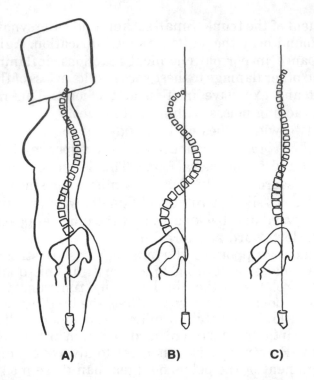

A)   **B)**   **C)**

Fig. 80—How you stand does affect your backache. Inside every patient with backache is a spine that's waging war with the forces of gravity. The angle of your spinal curves determine how you adapt to the constant downward "pull" on the frame by gravity. When posture is evenly balanced A) there are no points of weakness in the spine and muscles are not unnecessarily contracted. You are balanced in relation to gravity. You can determine this by allowing a plumb line to fall from your ear to your ankle. If you're allowing the pelvis, abdomen and shoulders to sag downward and forward B) the plumb line falls in back of its normal position. This off-center alignment means there is an anterior (forward) and downward sag in your framework which causes strain in the back muscles and ligaments. Figure C) shows the effect of a too rigid spine, a "military" posture, which also stretches muscles and ligaments which attach to the front part of the body. The normal curves will be lost following severe back strain. D) This is correct posture; it projects an enthusiastic inner-self confindence and feeling of the well-adjusted personality. E) Demonstrates the dejection and depression forthcoming from excessive laxness in muscles plus posture habits which allow the head to fall "forward" of the normal erect and desirable body stance.

222

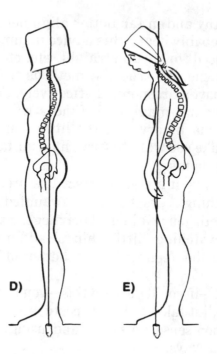

D)   E)

"When you get a few sprains in the knees, especially a clipping injury from the side, you've had it—your days with the team are numbered." He wasn't laughing as he said this.

Sprain has terminated the playing contract of many pros from the ranks of football, baseball, basketball and other competitive areas where players rely upon the integrity of the major joints for their living. It also ends the employment of many construction workers, truckers and iron workers.

A sprain results from diverse causes, many you no longer control or can avoid, the past injuries. However, you can prevent further damage by adopting good postural habits. Ten minutes a day lifting and pushing five pound dumbbells will help your upper trunk stay

223

fit and healthy and in far better alignment.

You've probably heard this advice innumerable times since childhood, to sit up straight, etc. etc. But, if you suffer backache, it's true the methods tried upon you failed, you haven't responded effectively. Consequently, your problem has magnified. Find a way to penetrate inside your machinery, get the little men turning the cranks to make you want to straighten up, take the strain off suffering joints.

Go for it! Give it a try. "Perfect Posture," as much as perfect anything . . . especially the vaunted perfection of "10" . . . is both your right and privilege. Experience the miracle of watching "little things" add up to personal satisfaction, the feeling you're better off today than yesterday.

Keep at it—if you'll only do this—you'll improve your backache. All it takes is better posture, stretching exercises, common-sense nutrition and using your body in less stressful ways.

One final consideration deserves mention.

Awkward posture is the outward extension of your inner self . . . it's body language that shouts things about you to everyone within listening distance. What you say with your body turns people on or off . . . especially a spouse, lover, employer or someone you wish will get the "right" impression of you in the quickest time.

Posture and strain go together, so expect gross postural defects to return nothing better than a backache, plus the same personal rejection you'd expect from wearing hair-rollers and ragged cut-offs to the Senior Prom.

ARTHRITIS ISN'T A FATAL DISEASE

There are many forms and many causes of arthritis, some of which cripple severely, and other types which result simply from biological wearing out of supporting tissues (Fig. 81).

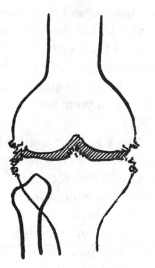

Fig. 81—Example of arthritic deposits in the knee. Authorities believe injury can be responsible for cracks in the cartilage lining the bones at joints, allowing fibrous tissue to infiltrate the joint. With other mineral substances intermixing within the crack an osteophyte (spur) is created which can irritate surrounding tissues. These stony deposits may occur in the vertebrae and actually build a bridge between two vertebra, performing a "natural fusion."

The infectious, rheumatoid type is not under consideration in this book. However, I have dealt with hundreds of patients who have figuratively "died" from having a doctor tell them they had "arthritis."

"Nothing can be done for it, you'll just have to live with it." This is probably the cruelest phrase a person can hear. The worst thing about this phrase is—it is not the truth, written in cement or produces any knee-jerk among the health professionals who use chiropractic procedures or physical medicine to restore arthritic individuals to a functional, productive and happy style of life.

There is much you can do to restore movement to degenerated joints through regular stretching movements of the involved parts. "Use it or lose it" must be your slogan to live by to rebuild strength in atrophied or flaccid muscles. A change in present nutritional insight and attitudes must motivate you to order a baked potato rather than french fries with ketchup. You must respect your body's metabolic needs at the expense of bad habits which add pounds to an already overburdened framework.

You must talk to professional counselors, who can lead you toward less stressful reactions to the strangling and abrasive problems occupying space in your personal or occupational environment.

Of course you don't *die* die when you hear you've got arthritis, but this pronouncement is so closely allied with fear that, learning about your condition, a cycle of depression and withdrawal starts which amounts figuratively to cashing in your remaining chips.

Forget your chronological age! Concentrate on a new start in life based upon your biological capabilities. Start an exercise program of walking—even around the block—and slowly progress with pleasant forms of physical rebuilding, like square dancing, jazzercize, bicycling, skipping rope, swimming, and other organized activities sponsored by local communities, the Y, Senior Citizen clubs, and the parks and recreation department in your city. These are usually free or involve minimal fees and are available to everyone.

The stretching exercises in this book, in addition to a short walk, will make you want to live and love, not feather a mortician's nest. Make it your goal to get involved with people, events, relatives and other forms of outgoing activities. People do need people.

Take a "what do you care" attitude if I'm not the best volunteer on the block—at least, I'm available, willing and ready.

PROBLEMS OF THE SPINAL DISC

Even the hint of a "disc problem" by a doctor and a large segment of society immediately recall horror stories they've heard. Surgery is the next step, they imagine . . . and the possibility of a future confined to a wheel chair.

Surgery is one form of last-resort therapy and sometimes is necessary for disc injury, however, it is not the only method available to repair a damaged intervertebral disc. And, only in a small percentage of cases—an unusually small percentage, at that—is surgery indicated over proper conservative treatment, based upon the reliable opinion of outstanding practitioners in the chiropractic and orthopedic professions.

Actually, thousands of patients at the Gonstead Clinic, Mt. Horeb, Wisconsin, have recovered from a diagnosis of disc pathology without surgery. Treatment here consists of specific chiropractic adjustments, the methods researched and developed by the founder, the late Dr. Clarence Gonstead.

Several thousand progressive chiropractors have attended educational seminars at the Gonstead Clinic. Here they study and keep abreast of modern techniques proven successful in returning patients with troublesome disc involvements to their former functional mode of living.

With an internal nucleus which moves within a semi-fluid media in response to foreward, backward and lateral bending, the spinal disc is a tough, fibrous, yet partially pliable, pad which separates the individual vertebra. It's normal shock-absorbing-like qualities can be impaired from breaks in its outer ring due to injury. A partial or total rupture—or disc herniation—causes loss in its natural heighth, bringing opposing vertebrae closer together, usually with painful results. Pressure on the lumbar disc is typically accompanied by pain referred to the sciatic nerve and the patient experiences sharp discomfort along the distribution of this nerve in the low back, buttocks, down the back of the thigh and calf, ending in the foot or toes. This pain may be exaggerated by coughing, sneezing or laughing (the Valsalva effect).

Both Drs. Doug and Alex Cox, the present directors of the Gonstead Clinic, studied under Dr. Gonstead several years before his death.

In response to my request for one case which typified their thousands of cases at the clinic, they chose the following:

A 36-year old professional football player was facing sudden retirement due to his physical condition, diagnosed as deteriortation of the disc at the third to fifth lumbar levels, accompanied by rupture and herniation of the fifth lumbar disc, sciatica and low back pain.

This individual not only was relieved of pain, he was back in the defensive lineup for three more years. Although now retired by choice, he is still an active athlete, running daily and aggressively pursuing a business career.

His treatment consisted entirely of methods utilized at

228

the clinic. No surgery was performed.

The Williams exercise of lying on the back and pulling the knees onto the chest to relieve disc pain is not recommended by Gonstead doctors. This exercise is the equivalent of bending over to touch the toes, it puts strain on the disc, rather than relieve it.

Dr. Alex Cox suggests instead what he terms the "Power Walk" exercise, taking long strides while tightening the abdominal muscles. Jogging is not desirable, however, one can sprint as far as comfortable and then walk back to the starting place. Sit-up exercises are also detrimental to a disc problem as the action of this exercise is identical to forward bending and increases the disc pressure. A sit-up, says Dr. Cox, is the equivalent of bending over and picking up a 50-pound load.

Spinal imbalance puts a load on the disc. This is the most frequent cause for disc irritation, as either the front or back portion of the disc receives an extra amount of compressive force when the vertebra above and below presses upon it as a result of this unequal load. Rather than being in their normally level horizontal position, corners of both vertebra are squeezing the life and resiliency from the helpless disc. Also, excessive backward movement of the disc creates a kink or bend in the posterior (back) longitudinal ligament, which is richly endowed with pain fibers. Additionally, alteration in the normal disc positions irritate the roots of spinal nerves with painful consequences.

EXERCISES THAT BENEFIT EVERYONE

Many times my back patients will ask, "Isn't there

some exercises I can do to get rid of this back problem?" There is and there isn't.

The same patient may consider his present difficulty as a "sudden" event, it just "happened." This thinking is akin to believing a heart attack is "sudden." A back pain—or a heart pain—doesn't happen suddenly to someone over thirty, it builds up over the years.

You may "break down" when your body parts cry "Enough of this strain! I can't take another pound of intolerance." That's when you experience back pain or acute problems.

A heart attack means the destruction which has occurred slowly during former years has reached its limits ... it can no longer stand the pressure. It reacts violently and tragically. But, the evidence found by the pathologist is seldom the unexplainable explosion of healthy tissue. Tissue destruction is the result of many years of inappropriate physiological behavior in tandem with a normal physical reaction to stressful conditions.

So, in answer to the patient's question about exercise, if you are presently suffering as a result of body misuse, further exercise is like practicing the wrong notes on the scale to become a good piano player ... the longer and harder you try, the worse you get.

Exercises should be performed to strengthen the particular weak areas associated with your specific condition. From this, it is obvious that performing certain exercises can further injure your body with movement which aggravates an already painful zone.

You can safely practice movements which have a stretching action on the muscles, ligaments and tendons. These tend to free the joints of the restriction against non-specific exercising.

Exercise should specifically strengthen the muscles which support the spine, the long, *spinae erectors* of the back and the upper and lower abdominals in the front of your body. Another important muscle, the *Psosas*, is frequently involved in backache, and it too, should be stretched and, when healed, exercised to regain additional function.

Swimming is not for everyone, especially the crawl stroke, which hyperextends the low back muscles and increases back pain in the lumbar area. Everyone can benefit from the weightless movements associated with the pool by just moving their body in all directions, without going beyond the point of pain or an inward sensation of resistance.

Side-bending exercises will help overcome a lateral curve in the back. Easy head-ups will improve abdominal strength. Pelvic tilting, lying or standing against a wall, will decrease a strain-producing bow in the low-back. Chest expanding exercises will help reduce the hump-like projection of the mid-back (kyphosis). Retracting the chin backward will eliminate a forward head carriage, which leads to downward sloping of the shoulders (and eventually shoulder and arm pain, numbness and tingling). Maintaining the knees in a slight forward bending attitude will correct a troublesome "back bending" in the knees and lessen the painful consequences of hamstring tightness and possibly sciatica. Replacing worn shoes will stabilize postural balance and reduce strain from several points of the body, even in the neck and head. Being fitted with corrective devices in the shoes to off-set anatomical defects, a short-leg or support for flat-feet, will improve general body balance.

Shedding extra pounds will take the strain from the

lower mid-back, caused by forward sag of the abdomen. It will also allow organs to maintain their intended positions within the body, not sag downward and create additional problems in digestion or elmination.

While some of these remedies are not "exercise," it should be considered that all movement is exercise, consequently, the more effectively you use your body, the more structurally perfect you are, the more activities performed by your body will benefit you, not harm you by increasing potentially destructive processes.

Your doctor must understand your condition to recommend specific exercises for your specific condition. Work with him and achieve your goal.

There is one exercise you can do without increasing damage. Walking. Walking with both arms swinging, drinking in the details of your surroundings while concentrating on an erect, proper posture.

You must have several ideas by now of what's wrong with you. Keep your faults plainly in mental view—not in a guilty sense—but accepting certain existing facts and making an effort to correct them. Study the perfect model. Get a feel for making positive corrections.

Go for it! And say "Bye Bye" to Backache.

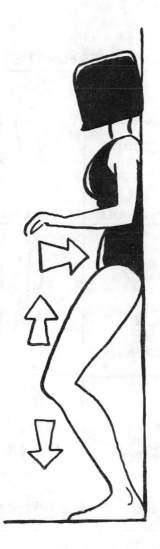

Fig. 82—Pelvic Tilt exercise. Stand against a wall and allow your body to slide up and down, keeping the low back flat against the wall. This exercise strengthens the front leg muscles and gives you the right feel for squatting movements. Start slowly and gradually increase the depth of bending. Don't force movement against pain. Allow yourself to gradually increase number of times you can repeat this exercise without experiencing muscle soreness or fatigue.

GOOD WARMUP EXERCISES FOR THE FEET AND LEGS

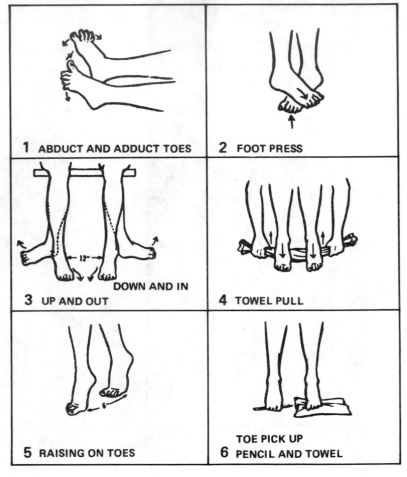

1 ABDUCT AND ADDUCT TOES

2 FOOT PRESS

DOWN AND IN

3 UP AND OUT

4 TOWEL PULL

5 RAISING ON TOES

TOE PICK UP
6 PENCIL AND TOWEL

Fig. 83—Move the ankles, feet and toes slowly through these exercises. Stretching exercises should be done in a relaxed manner. They are designed to make you feel better, so do them at a pace that suits you.

(Courtesy of the Foot Book, Harry F. Flacac, D.P.M., World Publications, Mt. View, CA).

234

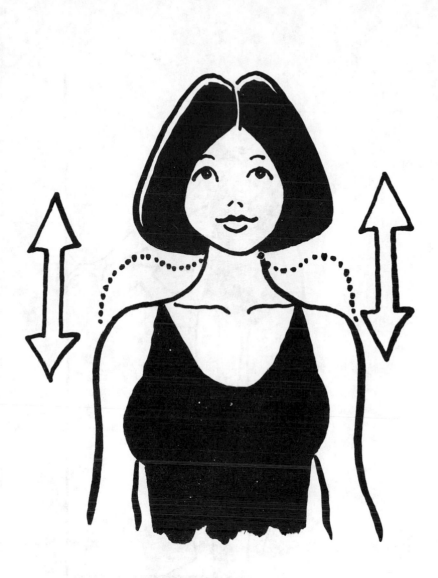

Fig. 84—Shoulder and scapula flexibility exercises. Shrugging the shoulders upward and downward moves the joints and associated tissues in the shoulder, clavical and scapula areas. To retrain the scapula from an outward projection, pull the shoulders backward while pushing the chest upward and forward. The scapula should not stick out. or protrude from the back.

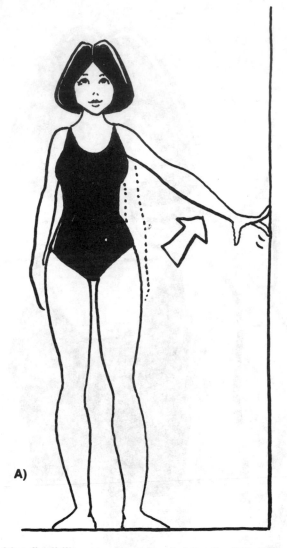

A)

Fig. 85—Shoulder flexibility can be extended by "walking up the wall." A) Face the wall and start your arm walk, while slowly turning your body B) until it reaches a right angle with the wall. Don't allow the entire shoulder joint to rise, it must remain level for this exercise to be effective. Constant practice will add flexibility to the several bones which form the "shoulder" joint.

236

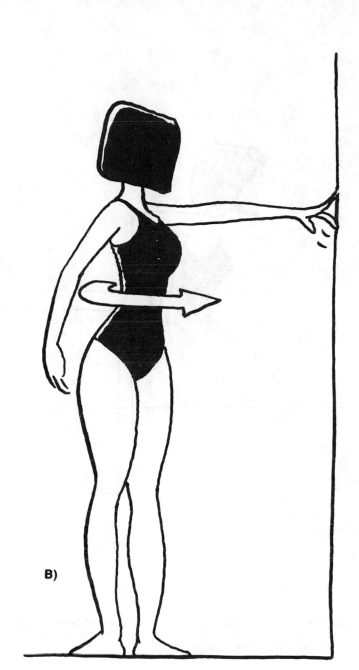

B)

237

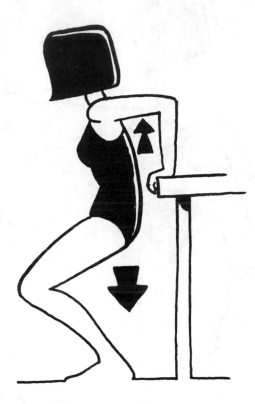

Fig. 86—This exercise strengthens muscles used in bending backward. Practice lowering yourself slowly into a deep knee bend with arms supported on a table behind you.

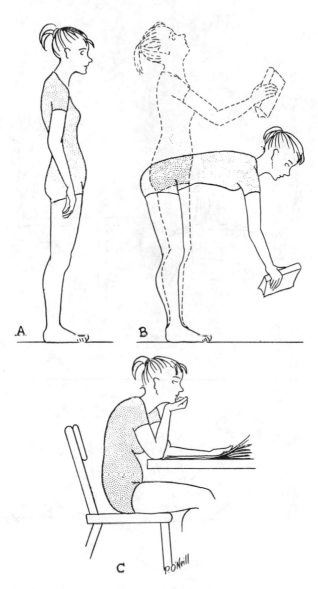

Fig. 87—Common postural attitude and misuse of body mechnaics.
A) Drooping shoulders B) Stooping C) Unusual "table posture"—
chin on hand.

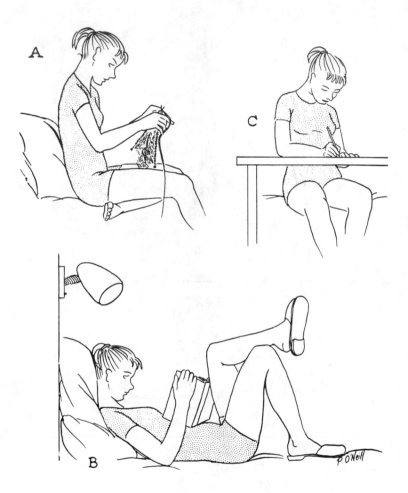

Fig. 88—Posture which strains the neck. A) Knitting or sewing B) Reading in bed C) Writing

(Figs. 87 and 88 courtesy of Cervical Syndrome, Ruth Jackson, M.D., Charles C Thomas, Springfield, Ill).

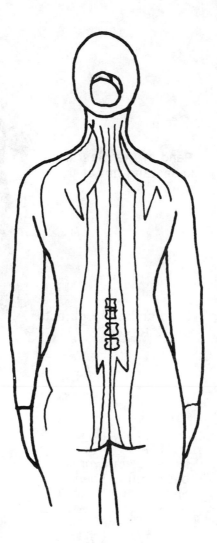

Fig. 89—The vertical lines in the back represent the Chinese Meridians which carry a flow of energy throughout the body. Acupuncturists and those who simulate this treatment with pressure, rather than penetrate the skin, stimulate or inhibit given points along these meridians to cause relief of pain. This form of treatment is graphically described in the book Acupressure, Acupuncture Without Needles by J.V. Cerney, D.P.M., published by Cornerstone Library, New York.

DO　　　　　　　　　　　　　　**DON'T**

Bend at the hips and
knees and not at the
waist.

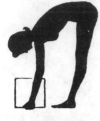

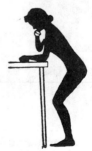

Hold and carry objects
close to you.

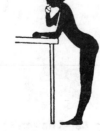

Never bend over with-
out bending knees
and tucking buttock
under.

242

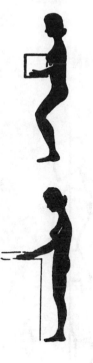

Keep back rounded as you return to standing from squat.

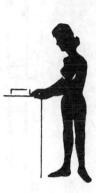

Always face your work and turn by pivoting your feet first.

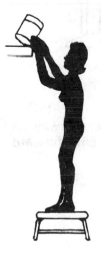

Keep buttock tucked under as you reach. Use a stool and avoid unnecessary reaching.

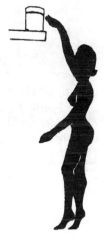

243

DO   **DON'T**

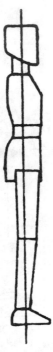

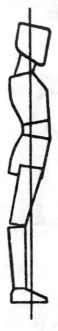

Stand tall with chin
in. Back flat, pelvis
tucked under and
knees relaxed.

Don't stand with
stiff knees, sway-
back or chin forward.

244

A P P E N D I X

PRODUCTS AVAILABLE TO
RELIEVE AND PREVENT BACKACHE

According to estimates of the federal government, the American public spends over $ 287 billion annually on their health. Can you guess what percentage pays for recovering from illness, versus the amount spent to prevent ill health?

I don't know the answer. Logic tells me it makes sense to invest a modest amount — at least — in yourself to stay well, active and pain-free.

The health marketplace bulges with products to keep you feeling fit...equipment to tone muscles, improve sluggish circulation, invigorate heart and lungs, build physical endurance and stamina for better posture and function of vital organs.

Cost-wise, these products have equal merit with so-called "health" insurance, used only when you're unhealthy. A means to prevent ill health proves far less expensive in the long run. Certainly, it's thousands times more exciting, relaxing and rewarding.

If your life is coupled to uncommon stress, counter-productive activity is a necessity. If you sit for long periods, additional back support is a must to overcome low back strain. Every back deserves a good mattress and a proper pillow for a comfortable night's rest. Your feet function best with good shoes.

A directory of health building products is provided for your inspection. Use it to find convenient, simple and inexpensive ways to benefit your health, overcome problems...things you can and should do to stay healthy.

245

The BACK-HUGGAR
A LOW BACK SUPPORT CUSHION

This back support cushion was developed by Dr. John Fiore, a chiropractor with 27 years clinical experience with problems affecting the spinal column.

Called the BACK-HUGGAR, this cushion combines proven scientific principles with a firm understanding of problems associated with the lumbar region.

The cushion is designed to shape the back to the natural curves of the spine to reduce unnecessary pain and stress. The diagrams show how ordinary support cushions offer no lateral support while the BACK-HUGGAR gives **circumferential support,** forcing discs in **both** forward and medial direction.

BACK-HUGGAR   **ORDINARY SUPPORT**

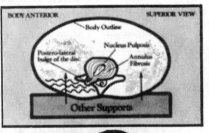

The BACK-HUGGAR gives support to the back to relieve stress and strain. It is especially useful while driving, working or at home.

It is designed to ease back strain associated with sitting for long periods, making almost any seat more comfortable.

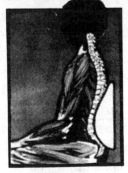

THE BACK-HUGGAR —
Developed By A Chiropractor To Ease
Common Low Back Pain

It takes but a few hours' time seated in a car or chair to realize that the "comfort" design leaves something to be desired. Often, the spine is forced into unnatural positions which can cancel nature's "shock-absorbing" feature, especially in the lower back.

This lumbar fatigue may eventually create a dull, irritating pain; the spine is distorted, and over a period of time this constant squeeze and distortion can create serious back problems.

Thousands of people have found the practical answer to comfort is the amazing BACK-HUGGAR. Developed by a Chiropractic physician, BACK-HUGGAR gets right to the cause and eliminates spinal pressure. With the BACK-HUGGAR in place the spine is allowed to follow its natural curve. It literally "hugs" the lower back and provides seating comfort in your car or at home, and is especially beneficial for people with back problems.

BACK-HUGGAR'S design is the result of years spent in testing and development. The comparatively simple design has one great advantage: It works!

"We traveled over 6000 miles and I can honestly say that I have never had anything that gave me such comfort on a trip. The 'HUGGAR' is great..."

That's the opinion of Dr. A.R. Helveston of Clinton, Tennessee. Dr. Fred Maisel in Gary, Indiana, wrote:

"...heard from the patient who drove to Miami Beach with the last cushion received and he says it was unbelievably comfortable. And he is a man with an aching lower lumbar area."

For more information write:
CONTOUR COMFORT CO., 7240 Lem Turner Rd., Jacksonville, Florida 32208.

INVERSION THERAPY

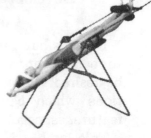

INVERSION — Reached at full open position for maximum decompression.

INCLINED/OSCILLATION — With arms above head you control the angle of inversion.

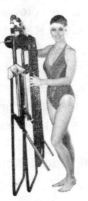

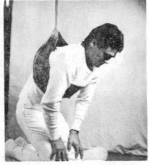

THE BACK BUBBLE

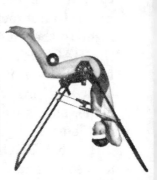

STORAGE — Store in a matter of seconds by folding into position shown.

PELVIC TRACTION — This optional feature allows traction in fixed position.

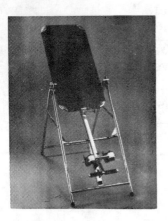

the BACK BUBBLE

Let your own body weight apply spinal traction to overcome stress of gravity. The BACK BUBBLE'S inflatable harness and unique spring assembly gives a feeling of weightlessness. Use it upright, inverted or semi-prone as a valuable tool for a pain-free back.

248

VIEW YOUR BACK PAIN
FROM A DIFFERENT ANGLE...

Life in the upright position means a daily struggle against the forces of gravity which pull and compress our bodies downward. This constant pressure can influence the healthy tissues of the body, especially the vertebral discs and other soft tissue parts which make up your spinal support system.

How can the effects of gravity — which many authorities believe contribute to back pain and heart trouble — be successfully overcome?

By hanging up-side-down in a comfortable fashion for even a few minutes each day.

With the use of an inversion machine users can invert their positions to gain relaxation, increase blood flow to the brain, help drain the lymphatic system, utilize traction to relieve pressures on spinal segments, reduce strain from lubricating areas of the joint facets and improve positioning of internal organs.

For more information about the many advantages of home care for bad backs with inversion therapy, consult your doctor.

AIR FLOTATION SLEEP SYSTEM — THE AIR BED FOR TOTAL COMFORT

Ask anyone familiar with backache what gives them the greatest relief from pain and you'll probably be told, "A good night's sleep."

Such a simple remedy isn't always as simple as it sounds, even in this age of high technology.

The pressure points which irritate your spinal column may result from a mattress suffering from the "Toos"... it's too lumpy, sagging, short, hard, narrow, soft or the innersprings gouge your sore muscles like a cattle prod.

The logical solution — sleeping on a bed of air — to an irritating problem like a backache is almost too simplistic to be accepted. Nevertheless, the effectiveness of an air bed to reduce distress from aching and cramping muscles is reported by happy people who have switched to the air bed.

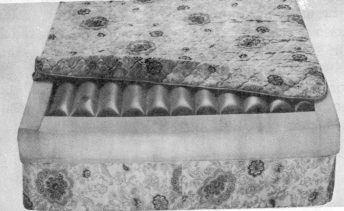

Imagine, a sleeping surface that's adjustable to your intimate dimensions of personal comfort — merely by adding air for firmness or releasing air for downy pleasure.

Medical researchers, who measured pressure on various parts of the back and heel, found the air bed allowed for the most efficient pressure distribution compared to ten other sleeping surfaces, including water beds and conventional mattresses.

FOR ADDITIONAL INFORMATION, WRITE:

AIR BEDS, INC. 2082 Zanker Road, San Jose, Ca. 95131

408-279-1444

Doctors laughed when we said we could help their patients.

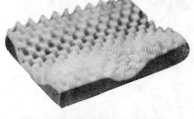

PROPILLOW®

DOCTOR-DESIGNED NECK SUPPORT PILLOW

Now doctors are smiling at their bottom line benefits from usage of the classic PROPILLOW from ProTech. The PROPILLOW* offers patented, multi-layer neck support with the famous "neck cradle" protection for the 30% of patients who suffer from aggravating neck and shoulder pain. No more punching your ordinary pillow into shape to get comfortable. PROPILLOW provides proper sleep posture now recognized to help prevent morning stiffness and pain. And what's more, after 2 years the PROPILLOW has cured sagging pillow patient benefits.
*Doctor-designed.

NECK-SHAPE™

TRI-LEVEL NECK SUPPORT PILLOW

NECK-SHAPE is new! Sensibly priced and designed for comfort, it's the newest shape of a good night's sleep from ProTech. NECK-SHAPE's "tri-level" design provides comfort and neck support in both back and side-sleeping positions. So helpful to the 55-70% of you who sleep on your side. Run your hand over the bonded surface of convoluted foam and feel the dozens of tiny "hills and valleys." This surface is the touch of genius which keeps customers coming back for ProTech products. Both pillows made from 100% polyurethane foam with zip-off protectors.

Talk to your Doctor, call or write today.

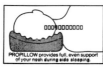

PROPILLOW provides full, even support of your neck during side sleeping.

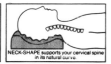

NECK-SHAPE supports your cervical spine in its natural curve.

ProTechPacific

1221 Andersen Drive
San Rafael, CA 94901
(800) 554-5541
U.S. Patent No. 4320543

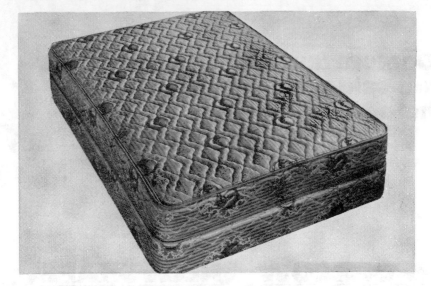

ChiroTonic Sleep Set

Do you get plenty of exercise and watch what you eat to stay in good health?

Well, like exercise and nutrition, a good night's sleep is also essential for good health . . . feeling good every day starts with a good night's sleep.

The new Restonic ChiroTonic mattress is designed for people concerned about getting maximum body support needed for a good night's sleep. The ChiroTonic is the only mattress with an insulator for extra support you can feel.

Restonic products are rated by Consumer Report among the nation's top five best sleep systems.

There are many imitators, but only one Restonic Chiro-Tonic . . . sample it in the dealer's showroom and you won't accept anything less than the best for wonderful, lasting back comfort.

Restonic Corporation, Inc.
101 No. Wacker Dr., Chicago, ILL 60606

THE FOUNDATION FOR A HEALTHY BACK

Good physical hygiene requires a stable foundation for upright posture . . . both night and day.

At night, good posture support comes with sleeping on a suitably firm, comfortable and generous mattress with sturdy coil springs in the box foundation.

During the day chiropractors are on their feet most of the time. Is it any wonder they value shoes which support all the architecture above the ankle? A good foundation means wearing well constructed shoes to maintain balanced support.

Ask your doctor what to do about a short leg. A heel lift or insert may be required for body balance. or, you may require shoe reconstruction.

For maximum stbility, I recommend the ROOTS NATURAL FOOTWARE both for walking and for the user who is on his feet a good portion of the day. Look at the construction—it's made to give your body the foundation needed for a healthy back.

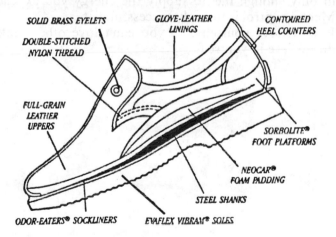

253

SUMMARY:

FOUR CARDINAL RULES
FOR A HEALTHY BACK

1. You've learned how imbalance—poor posture—turns a normal back into a backache. How even a slight malalignment of the spine (a subluxation) results in muscle weakness, cramping, and pain when you twist, turn, sit or lie down . . . even in locations and organs distant from where it hurts. The solution lies in correcting your present problems of poor posture, sleeping on a soft, lumpy mattress and wearing poorly fitted, non-supportive shoes. Create your own environment at work with back supporting chairs and non-straining foundation for standing long hours.

2. Walk daily. Build up those weak, tired and sagging back and stomach muscles. Stretch the tight ligaments and muscles.

3. Learn all you can about nutrition. Avoid overeating, take in only enough fuel to supply the energy you expend daily. Mental control is the only successful diet.

4. Finally, love yourself . . . you can't love others unless you do. Believe in yourself.